THE RIDER'S
FITNESS GUIDE

to a

Better Seat

THE RIDER'S FITNESS GUIDE

to a

Better Seat

JEAN-PIERRE HOURDEBAIGT, LMT

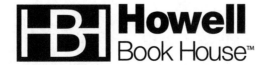

Copyright © 2008 by Jean-Pierre Hourdebaigt. All rights reserved.
Photos copyright Stacey Killmaier.

Howell Book House
Published by Wiley Publishing, Inc., Hoboken, New Jersey

For general information on our other products and services or to obtain technical support please contact our Customer Care Department within the U.S. at (800) 762-2974, outside the U.S. at (317) 572-3993 or fax (317) 572-4002.

Wiley also publishes its books in a variety of electronic formats. Some content that appears in print may not be available in electronic books. For more information about Wiley products, please visit our web site at www.wiley.com.

Library of Congress Cataloging-in-Publication Data:
Hourdebaigt, Jean-Pierre.
   The rider's fitness guide to a better seat / Jean-Pierre Hourdebaigt.
      p. cm.
   ISBN: 978-0-470-13743-7 (pbk.)
   1. Horsemanship.   I. Title.
   SF309.H685 2008
   798.2'3—dc22

Printed in the United States of America

10 9 8 7 6 5 4 3 2

Book design by Lissa Auciello-Brogan and Erin Zeltner
Cover design by José Almaguer
Book production by Wiley Publishing, Inc. Composition Services

TABLE OF CONTENTS

LIST OF FIGURES

PREFACE

Congratulations! You have made a wonderful investment in your future by purchasing *The Rider's Fitness Guide to a Better Seat.*

This book is a complete study of the ideal rider seat and of the muscle groups utilized when sitting properly in the saddle. In time, the knowledge gained from this book will allow you to increase your control over your core muscles, which will vastly improve your riding skills resulting in a finer and effortless execution.

After you have satisfied your curiosity and familiarized yourself with the content by scanning the book, proceed with studying the strengthening exercises and stretches. I recommend you read the book once from cover to cover. Then go through it again, but this time you should actually practice the exercises and even take notes if you wish. This method will help you fully absorb the material presented.

This book was written in a simple language for everyone to understand. Confusion or an inability to learn most often results when the reader does not understand the text. If the material presented becomes confusing, then go back and reread it to make sure you understand every word.

The content of this book is presented in an orderly sequence to build up your knowledge of body care. You can't progress in your education with parts of your knowledge being unclear because this would adversely affect your riding performance. To make the most of this material you need to be willing to set aside enough time to read the entire book and also develop a schedule for incorporating the exercises into your daily routine.

Having a busy life doesn't leave much free time for hobbies or studies. For your studies, 15- to 20-minute study sessions work best. Studying is easier and faster if you work on little sections at a time rather than large chunks at once.

Good habits are the key to success. To get a good start, spend a minimum of one session per day, three days per week, reading this book. Be creative and stay focused. The few moments you spend each day reading this book are a small price to pay for the knowledge, happiness, and success that will be yours when you start feeling stronger and more in control of your riding.

At first, this entire program may seem to be a rather large task to undertake. But remember, the knowledge you are developing will stay with you for a lifetime. Take it one step at a time, and before you know it you will have absorbed a lot and you will feel pretty confident. Persist and you will succeed. Exercise every day!

A part of making this learning process a fun experience is to give yourself rewards as you complete each chapter of the book. Take yourself out to a movie or dinner, or buy yourself some new clothes. Enjoy the learning process. Relax, take lots of deep breaths, and smile. Do not forget to appreciate the learning curve you are going through. As you combine this material with your instincts as a horse person, you will soon feel stronger and more confident in your riding seat.

Jean-Pierre Hourdebaigt, LMT,
President of Massage Awareness, Inc.

ACKNOWLEDGMENTS

My sincere gratitude goes to all the riders and other professionals who have shared their stories with me, their needs and hopes, and, most important, their knowledge and feedback over the years. This life-sharing experience has been a source of inspiration to me.

For making this publication possible, I especially thank:

Brigitte Hourdebaigt, for making my life a beautiful experience every day.

Brigitte Hawkins, for taking beautiful pictures of my horse and me.

Stacey Killmaier, for her professional talent in taking the photos used in this book.

Julie-Anne and Xavier Staiger, for their modeling talents, patience, and enduring sense of humor.

INTRODUCTION

A good *seat*—that is, the manner of sitting on a horse and maintaining good balance—is vital to all riders because it ensures a good riding performance. Riding is a sport of harmony where the rider keeps rhythm with the horse. A good seat allows for better communication through your aids (such as legs, reins, and seat), which leads to a more harmonious and effortless contact with your horse, allowing him to work at his best. Otherwise, you end up spending a lot of energy constantly adjusting your balance and fighting gravity, a very tiring experience, in order to keep up with your horse's performance. To be *in tune* with your horse, you need to develop an *independent* seat, that is, a personal sense of balance without having to depend on the horse. In turn, a good seat will provide the horse with the security he needs to regain his natural balance at all gaits because he does not have to compensate for your uneven seat. Developing strong core body muscles (abdominals and back) will help you to achieve an independent seat and an independent application of the aids.

This book explains the essential characteristics of a good seat and provides a fitness program toward achieving it. If you want to improve your riding, you have to actually *practice* good riding techniques. You need to honestly assess whether you are willing to commit to this exercise program. Simply theorizing or speculating about your options is not enough. You need to find the time to strengthen your core muscles, which will improve your posture and give you a better seat. Becoming aware of the muscles responsible for a good seat will help you to focus on increasing the fitness and flexibility of these muscles. This will result not only in an overall better posture, but also in better stamina and sense of balance. In a more relaxed manner, you will better control any movements, leaning either sideways, forward, or backward to realign your center of gravity with the horse's center of gravity, influencing the horse to move effectively and without much effort.

Often riders say that the best way to develop "riding muscles" is to ride. That is true; however, it is not enough. The most obvious example is the rider's ability to sustain a sitting trot. The sitting trot is the most demanding aspect of riding, especially with a tall horse. Absorbing the horse's movement and going with the horse's flow requires core strength, a supple back, and overall fitness of the upper and lower body, as well as a healthy aerobic fitness, because maintaining a sitting trot can quickly cause a rider to huff and puff.

1

If the core muscles are not strong enough, the back muscles and the spinal structure will absorb the slack, which often results in a sore back. Also, if the rider lacks lower-back flexibility, his ride will be bumpy because he will be bouncing in the saddle, causing his lower back to become sore. The unabsorbed forces created by the bouncing have to go somewhere, so they usually end up in the lower legs, causing stiff ankles and losing the stirrups, and in the upper body, causing stiffness in the shoulders, the elbows to turn out, unsteady hands, and bobbing of the neck. Not a pretty sight! To maintain a proper seat at the sitting trot, a rider needs sufficient core muscle strength and overall fitness; otherwise, he will tire very easily, losing coordination and his seat.

It is your responsibility to develop your core muscles and to be fit if you want to fully enjoy riding. This book provides three exercise programs—beginning (10 days), intermediate (20 days), and advanced (ongoing/maintenance)—that will help you increase your control over a better seat. To maximize performance and to minimize the risk of injury, many top athletes, regardless of their chosen sport, use a cross-training approach to their training. For example, a long-distance runner will incorporate some swimming and weight training into his routine. This training strengthens core muscles, resulting in improved balance, strength, and endurance. This particular cross-training philosophy of working from the core is reflected in the selection of exercises that make up the various programs presented in this book.

This book contains information useful to all riders, both amateur and professional. It provides general anatomical knowledge of all the muscles involved in the seat and a comprehensive listing of strengthening exercises and follow-up stretches to put the rider in tune with his body. None of these exercises require any equipment and they can easily be performed anywhere. So you can maintain your fitness even when you are on the road.

If you practice these simple exercise programs, you will greatly increase your strength and stamina and improve your coordination within 30 days. And you will also have a better seat!

You will notice a physical difference in your body after just 10 days of exercise and by the end of the month you will have a new awareness of your body. The three exercise programs presented in this book will transform the way your body feels and performs. These simple exercises will help you develop greater body awareness, good posture, and an easy, graceful seat. Welcome to the beginning of your new riding experience. I hope this book will contribute to your success.

1

COMPONENTS OF A GOOD SEAT

The seat is the rider's primary and most important point of influence with the horse. The rider's weight in the seat and the pressure of his legs on the horse are considered the initial driving aids to determine the forward movement of the horse. The horse will immediately feel any movements initiated from the hips and/or legs. The arms and hands governing the reins are considered secondary aids, assisting in the regulation of movement and stabilizing the gait and the direction of the horse. When you are comfortable with your seat and legs, then you can relax your upper body. This posture allows you to be steadier with your hands and have a good contact with the horse's mouth via the bit.

DEVELOPING A GOOD SEAT

For a comfortable seat, the rider should sit with his back straight, centered and balanced in the seat, and only supported by the stirrups. The rider should allow his legs and arms to work independently from his torso.

The seat is the first area to develop if you want to enhance your riding experience. A good seat helps you with your balance while in motion regardless of the horse's gait. In order to attain a good seat, you need to develop strong *core muscles*, meaning strong abdominal and back muscles, which help you keep your balance much more easily. Keeping your abdominal muscles engaged, meaning slightly contracted, will allow you to relax the rest of your pelvic muscles; there should be no muscular stiffness in the pelvic area. Your inner thigh should rest against the saddle and the inside of your calf should rest against the horse's chest (barrel). Your feet should rest securely in the stirrups with the toes positioned nearly parallel to the horse's sides. Your seat should be

3

relaxed, with flexible hips, slightly bent knees, and supple ankles. This particular combination allows both legs to work as shock absorbers in order to better handle the horse's gait.

Also, strong core muscles help you integrate your pelvis and shoulder girdle so your torso and spine move in sync with the horse's gait. Your head should be balanced on the top of your shoulders and should not tilt forward or back. Keep your arms along the sides of your body with your forearms and hands relaxed. This upper torso position secures a good contact with the bit via the reins. Understand that you should not use the reins for support or balance, nor should you squeeze your legs against the horse's sides. These actions would interfere with the horse's movement and you would lose your seat.

The correct use of a good basic position that is centered, aligned, symmetrical, balanced, and relaxed creates an evenly conditioned body and prevents tension buildup and injuries. Physical fatigue during practices or training causes postural changes that make you use your legs and arms more. Keep in mind that when you are physically tired, you are mentally tired and you will start to make mistakes. Therefore, developing a good seat helps you save energy and seriously decreases the risk of making mistakes.

Becoming aware of the muscles involved and responsible for a good seat helps you understand the importance of developing core-muscle fitness and maintaining flexibility. This fitness will result in an overall better posture, leading to a more harmonious and effortless contact with your horse, allowing him to work at his best. The exercises presented in this book will help you improve your core strength, flexibility, agility, and economy of motion. Regular practice of these exercises also will help you alleviate back pain and other chronic ailments.

FINDING YOUR CENTER OF GRAVITY

When riding, you sit directly over the horse's center of gravity. If your center of gravity moves in sync with the horse's center of gravity, your ride becomes harmonious in all riding situations, whether the horse moves forward or engages in both upward and downward transition. Please take the time to observe the various riding disciplines in figure 1.1 to appreciate how the rider's center of gravity is always above the horse's center of gravity.

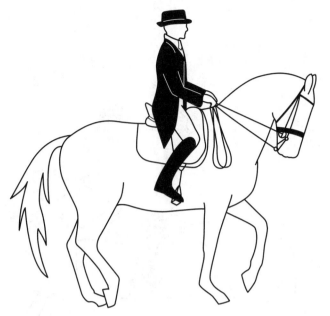

Dressage

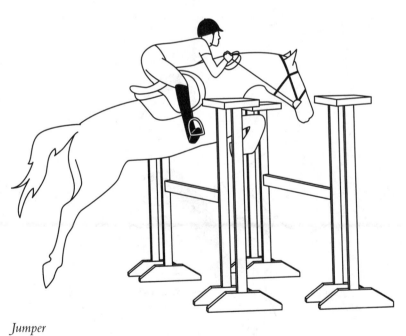

Jumper

Figure 1.1 Six riders with good seats.

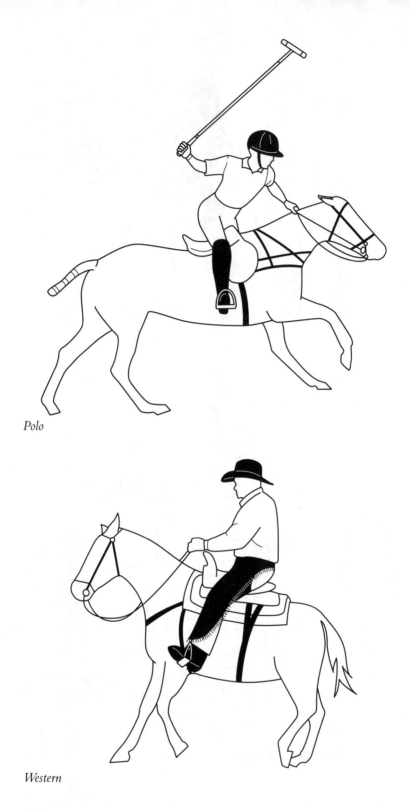

Polo

Western

Figure 1.1 Six riders with good seats (continued).

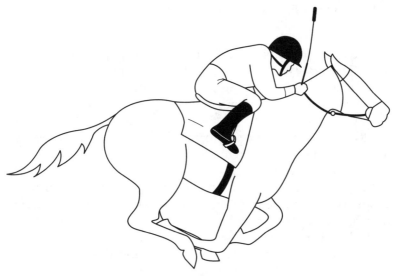

Racing

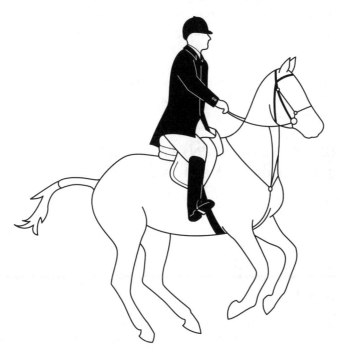

Hunt

Figure 1.1 Six riders with good seats (continued).

The *center of gravity* is that point where an object balances perfectly. The *line of gravity* is the line that passes from the body's center of gravity toward the center of the Earth.

In a human being standing in an upright position, the center of gravity can be found low in the pelvis, slightly above the second sacral vertebra, at about approximately 55 percent of a person's height. This point is located where the spine curves forward the most, as shown in figure 1.2.

Keep in mind that the center of gravity varies between males and females. A female has a larger pelvis, which results in her center of gravity lying slightly lower than in a male. It is only a minor detail, but worth mentioning.

A horse's center of gravity is located in mid-thorax at the level of the eighth rib, as shown in figure 1.3.

Riding over the horse's center of gravity in a relaxed manner allows you to gently control any movements by leaning sideways, forward, or backward to displace the alignment of the two centers of gravity, thereby influencing the horse effectively and without much effort.

The sooner you become aware of your center of gravity, the sooner you will reach that harmonious feeling with your horse. Developing strong core muscles will help you to feel your center of gravity.

FINDING YOUR CENTER OF GRAVITY: THE ROCKING EXERCISE

In most martial arts disciplines, discovering one's center of gravity is one of the first teachings, as it helps to build a solid foundation. The Rocking Exercise is used to help martial arts students discover their center of gravity. This very simple exercise will help you to discover and feel your own center of gravity, too.

Starting Position

Stand relaxed, arms at your sides, with your feet spread approximately at shoulder width so that you are standing solidly on your legs, which should be aligned with your hip joints. Your knees should be slightly bent. Keep your back straight throughout the entire exercise.

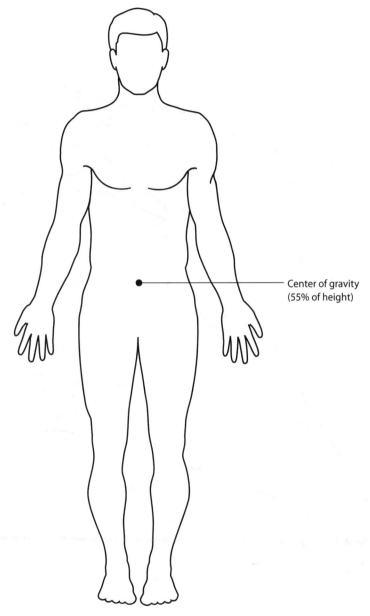

Center of gravity
(55% of height)

Figure 1.2 The human center of gravity.

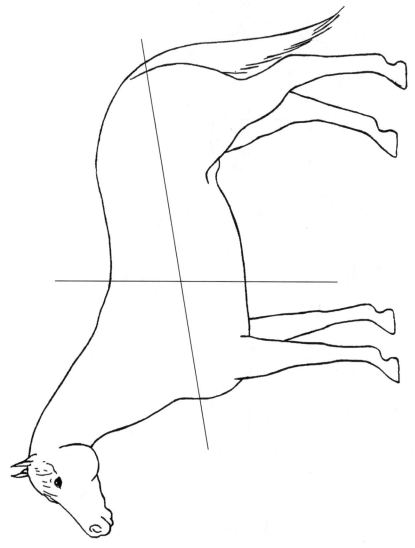

Figure 1.3 The equine center of gravity.

The Exercise

Slowly rock your body forward from your ankles until you feel your heels lifting and without losing your balance. Then rock backward in the same fashion until you feel your toes lifting off the ground, again without losing your balance. Repeat a few times until you are comfortable with your balance. Now, at the end of your last movement backward, when you reach the point where you feel the balls of your feet almost lifting off the floor, hold your position for one second. Feel the tension in your lower back, buttocks, and thighs.

Next, slowly move forward until the sensation of tension disappears. At that very point, you have reached your center of gravity. Stay there for a moment. Then twist your shoulders back and forth around the axis of your spine. This action will engage your core muscles and help you further define your center of gravity as you hold your posture.

I recommend you practice this exercise several times so that being aware of your center of gravity becomes almost second nature. The sooner you learn this technique, the sooner you will improve not only your riding seat, but your ability to do other kinds of physical exercise. Your center of gravity is also your center of energy, from which springs most of your hip and leg movements.

MAINTAINING YOUR BALANCE WITH THE HORSE

If an area of your body comes out of alignment, other areas will compensate in an effort to maintain a general sense of balance. The major areas of the body that can become misaligned when riding are the head, shoulders, back, and lower legs.

For example, when the head of the rider goes too far forward, the seat and torso move forward and the legs go too far back. The overall alignment is lost because the building blocks of your body are no longer supportive and in harmony with the horse's center of gravity. Leaning sideways, forward, or backward will displace the alignment of the two centers of gravity. Maintaining good alignment is essential in order to influence the horse effectively and without much effort.

The rider compensates in his shoulders, torso, back, and legs for misalignment in order to maintain his balance. The horse will also compensate for misalignment by shifting his weight to keep the rider's weight balanced comfortably over his center of gravity while maintaining his course. All of this compensation and realignment creates extra work for your body and will tire you and your horse out more quickly, leading to a less enjoyable ride for both of you. But if you maintain good physical fitness, you are much less likely to lose your balance and can therefore avoid compensation problems.

ACHIEVING SYMMETRY AND BALANCE IN RIDING

A good seat requires symmetry between the sides of your body. To quickly evaluate your own posture, stand in front of a full-length mirror. Observe if your body is symmetrical or lopsided. Ask yourself the following questions:

* Are my shoulders level?
* Are my hips and knees aligned?
* Are my toes facing straight ahead?

How do you rate? If your body shows some serious asymmetry, it might be time to consider contacting a physiotherapist or massage therapist to further assist you. A few good massage sessions will help you regain proper lateral symmetry. Remember that any asymmetry in the rider's body will affect the horse's training and muscular development. So, first address your posture before correcting your horse's posture.

Observing your overall balance while riding is very useful, too. If mirrors are available where you ride, you can evaluate if your body is evenly distributed on the horse by facing a mirror in the arena. Notice if the same areas of the body are level and if the stirrups are even. If no mirrors are available, have somebody take pictures of you or film you while you are riding.

Keep in mind that other factors can cause you to be off balance. An unbalanced saddle can be the cause. Also, a horse's own asymmetry can be a factor. Therefore, always make sure none of these factors are affecting your balance.

CONCLUSION

A good seat allows you to be relaxed, centered, aligned, symmetrical, and balanced. Developing strong core muscles creates an evenly conditioned body and prevents the buildup of tension and injuries, and reduces the incidence of mistakes.

But most important, a good seat allows you to work better from your center of gravity. This in turn helps you to align better with your horse's center of gravity. The secret of a harmonious ride is for the rider's center of gravity to move in sync with the horse's center of gravity, a position that should be maintained in all riding situations.

2

HUMAN ANATOMY

The human skeleton is made up of more than 206 bones and 500 muscles. This chapter presents an overview of the important bones and muscles that are used in the exercises presented later in this book. Familiarize yourself with these bones and muscles to better understand the purpose of the core muscle exercises.

A precise description of the human skeleton and musculature is beyond the scope of this book. For more information see the appendix, "Suggested Readings," for specific medical texts.

SKELETON

The human *skeleton* is the supporting structure of your body. It enables you to stand erect as well as accomplish various athletic and artistic endeavors. The skeleton is composed of 206 bones, distributed as follows:

❖ The *axial skeleton* (the skeleton of the trunk and head) consists of the spine, the skull, the hyoid bone, and the rib cage (including the sternum).

❖ The *appendicular skeleton* is comprised of the limbs (or appendages) of the body and includes the *upper extremities* (including the shoulder girdle) and the *lower extremities* (including the pelvic girdle).

❖ The bones that comprise the *upper extremities* include:

• The scapula and the clavicle, which form the shoulder girdle; and

• The humerus, radius, ulna, and carpus bones of the wrist, and the metacarpus and phalanges of the hand, which together form the entire arm.

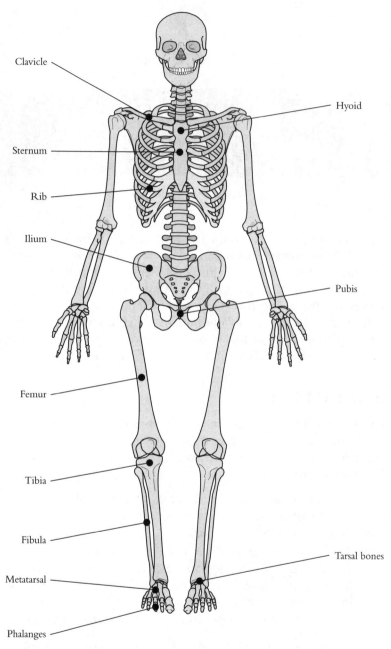

Clavicle

Hyoid

Sternum

Rib

Ilium

Pubis

Femur

Tibia

Fibula

Tarsal bones

Metatarsal

Phalanges

Figure 2.1 Anterior view of the major bones of the human skeleton.

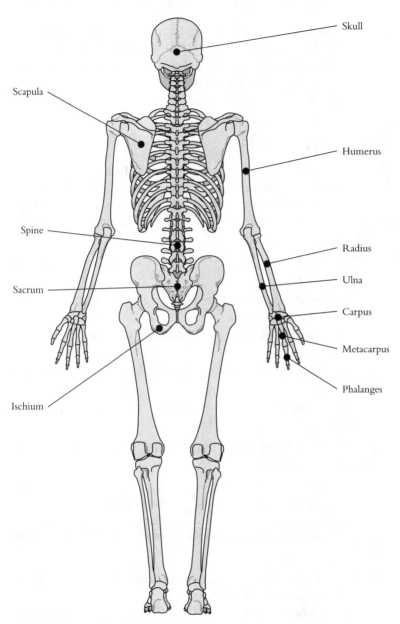

Figure 2.2 Posterior view of the major bones of the human skeleton.

❖ The bones that make up the *lower extremities* include:

  • The ilium, the pubis, the ischium, and the *sacrum* (five fused vertebrae), which form the pelvic girdle; and

  • The femur, tibia, and fibula; the tarsal bones of the ankle; and the metatarsal and phalange bones of the foot, which all together form the leg.

MUSCULATURE

This review of the human muscular system focuses only on the skeletal muscles. There are over 135 major skeletal muscles, which compose 40 to 50 percent of the body's weight. To simplify recognition of muscle functions, the skeletal muscles are classified into several categories. The main muscle categories are:

❖ The *abductor muscles,* which move a limb away from the midline of the body.

❖ The *adductor muscles,* which move a limb toward the midline of the body.

❖ The *extensor muscles,* which straighten a limb or the trunk at a joint.

❖ The *flexor muscles,* which bend a limb or the trunk at a joint.

❖ The *rotator muscles,* which rotate the involved bones at a joint.

This list contains all of the muscles that form the body's main skeletal muscle groups:

❖ *Arm muscles:* The deltoid, the biceps, the triceps, and the flexor and the extensor groups of the hand.

❖ *Back muscles:* The erector spinae group, the quadratus lumborum, the latissimus dorsi, and the neck extensor and flexor muscle groups.

❖ *Hip muscles:* The iliacus and the psoas (which make up the iliopsoas), and the gluteus.

❖ *Leg muscles:* The quadriceps, the hamstrings, the adductors, the flexors (the calf), and the extensors (the shins) of the foot.

❖ *Shoulder muscles:* The deep-seated rotator cuff muscle group, made up of the supraspinatus, infraspinatus, and subscapularis muscles (*not* shown on figures 2.3 through 2.5); the teres minor and major; the subclavius (also *not* shown on figures 2.3 through 2.5); and the pectorals.

❖ *Torso muscles:* The abdominals.

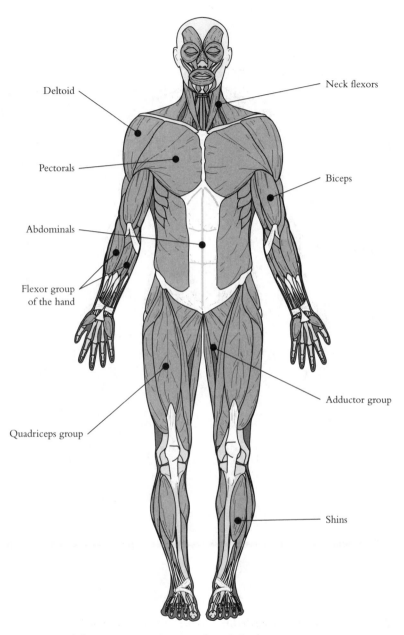

Deltoid

Pectorals

Abdominals

Flexor group
of the hand

Quadriceps group

Neck flexors

Biceps

Adductor group

Shins

Figure 2.3 The major anterior muscles of the human anatomy.

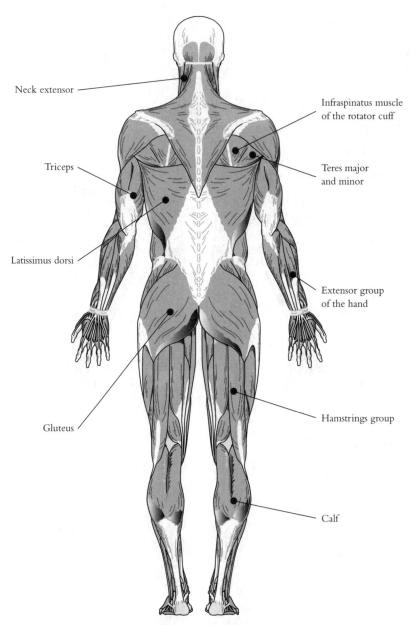

Neck extensor

Triceps

Latissimus dorsi

Gluteus

Infraspinatus muscle
of the rotator cuff

Teres major
and minor

Extensor group
of the hand

Hamstrings group

Calf

Figure 2.4 The major posterior muscles of the human anatomy.

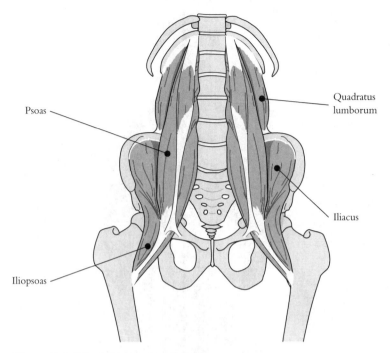

Figure 2.5 The hip muscles of the human anatomy.

Psoas

Quadratus
lumborum

Iliacus

Iliopsoas

THE CORE MUSCLES

The body's core muscles are considered great stabilizers of the lower back. The core muscles are comprised of the following two muscle groups:

1. The **back (erector spinae) muscle group** includes three major muscle bundles that run along your entire back from your neck to your lower back:

   • The *iliocostalis* (cervicis, lumborum, and thoracis sections)
   • The *longissimus* (capitis, cervicis, and thoracis sections)
   • The *spinalis* (capitis, cervicis, and thoracis sections)

2. The **abdominal muscle group** includes four muscles that run from your rib cage to your hips:

   • The *external oblique,* located on the sides and front of the abdomen (around your waist), is the most superficial muscle of the group and is responsible for twisting movements of the body. The muscle fibers run from the rib cage *down* toward the hipbone.

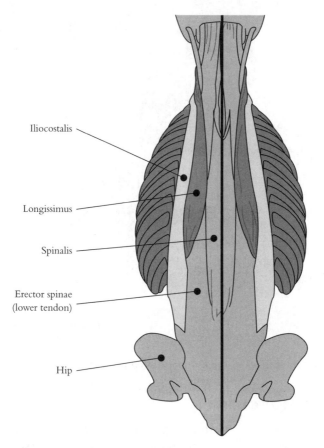

Figure 2.6 The core muscles of the back (erector spinae) muscle group.

- The *internal oblique* lies underneath the external oblique muscle and has the same function, but its fibers run in the opposite direction, running *up* from the hipbone toward the rib cage.
- The *rectus abdominis* is most often referred to as the "six-pack" muscle. This long muscle, located beneath the internal oblique muscle and extending from the sternum to the pubis, is responsible for bending the body forward (called the "anterior flexion" of the body).
- The *transversus abdominis* is the deepest muscle of the group. This muscle supports your back and provides stability and protection.

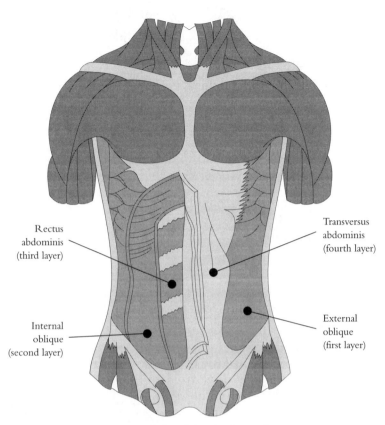

Rectus
abdominis
(third layer)

Transversus
abdominis
(fourth layer)

Internal
oblique
(second layer)

External
oblique
(first layer)

Figure 2.7 Anterior views of the abdominal muscle group.

3

PROPER BREATHING TECHNIQUES

Proper breathing allows you to maximize your performance when riding or practicing any of the exercises presented in this book. Breathing with your full lung capacity increases your oxygen input, resulting in more vitality. Furthermore, controlling your breathing is a great exercise to quiet and relax your mind. Controlled breathing helps you become focused and attentive, allowing you to constantly assess the sensations your body gives you. In yoga, it is said that if you use your full lungs, you use your full brain!

One of the most important factors of exercise is the proper development of the movements. To achieve the best results from exercise, an athlete must have the right mental attitude! So be relaxed and attentive to your exercise, and stay focused. You don't need to be serious and tense. Just relax, smile, and be aware of what you are doing. Do not let your mind wander. We have a tendency to let the left side of our brains dominate us, leading to rationalization and criticism, thereby reducing our perceptions and performance. By practicing relaxation techniques, you encourage the right brain to dominate, which allows you to have a more relaxed awareness of your environment, helping you to perform any task better. So take gentle and regular deep breaths, which will help you stay focused, yet relaxed. Breathing in this fashion lets both hemispheres of your brain function in harmony and this balance will enhance your perceptions. The resulting sense of calm will allow you to better feel and trust the sensory feedback received from your muscles and joints, improving the quality of your exercise. In the early stages of your exercise program, a very efficient way to develop this relaxed balance is to repeatedly take gentle, long breaths in the fashion presented on the following pages. With practice, these breathing techniques will become second nature.

Another benefit of proper breathing is that you get a great influx of oxygen. As you open your lungs during a full respiration, you boost your intake of oxygen and your evacuation of carbon dioxide. This is vital when exercising for long periods of time. A maximized oxygen level will contribute to your vitality, endurance, and efficiency of execution when exercising.

Tip: During your stretching routine, instead of counting seconds, consider taking deep breaths. For the average person, the "in" and "out" of a full and calm deep breath takes about 7 to 8 seconds. So just concentrate on taking deep breaths as you start each stretch. Take several deep breaths (five to ten) until the maximum stretching release is felt.

BREATHING MUSCLES

Proper breathing also comes from the diaphragm, not just the chest. Your shoulders should not lift when you inhale. Your upper chest should not rise until the very end of the inhalation.

Your main breathing muscle is your diaphragm muscle, located at the bottom of your rib cage. When you contract your diaphragm, it pulls the lungs down, drawing air in. As you relax the diaphragm, the lungs recoil, pushing the air out. The *intercostal muscles* and the *abdominal muscles* assist in the breathing-out phase.

TAKING A FULL BREATH

Normally, we breathe without giving it much thought and often only use a small portion of our total lung capacity. But you can improve your breathing awareness by learning to take a full breath. Start by taking a gentle but deep breath through the nose, filling the tops and sides of your lungs first, then the lower portion, stretching your stomach out. When your lungs are full, hold your breath a couple of seconds. Then release gently through the mouth, relaxing your stomach first, and completely expelling all the air from your lungs. Once your lungs are empty, hold your breath a couple of seconds.

Repeat the full breath cycle 3 to 5 times. This practice will help you stay focused, yet relaxed. During periods of tension, when showing your horse for example, practice the full breath several times until you feel calm.

Strengthening Breathing Exercises

The following two exercises will help you strengthen your breathing muscles so you can breathe more freely and efficiently, regardless of whether you are sitting or standing. Developing, or regaining, your full breathing ability is an important step that will benefit you for the rest of your life.

The Full Breath Exercise

You can practice this simple Full Breath Exercise to develop your awareness of how to take a full, deep breath.

Starting Position

Lie comfortably on your back with your legs straight, knees slightly bent, and arms relaxed by your side. Feel free to place pillows underneath your knees and your neck. Place a small light object on your belly, right over your navel, as shown in figure 3.1. You can use a jar of vitamins, a pot of cream, a tennis ball, or anything that fits and is not too heavy.

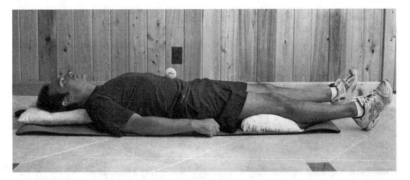

Figure 3.1 Full Breath Exercise, starting position.

The Exercise

Start the exercise by inhaling through your nose. As your lungs fill, progressively push your abdomen out, which will lift the object placed on your navel. Then, as you completely fill your lungs by expanding your sides and upper chest, push the object up as much as you can. At this point, you should see the object clearly. As you reach your limit, hold this position for a couple seconds, as shown in figure 3.2.

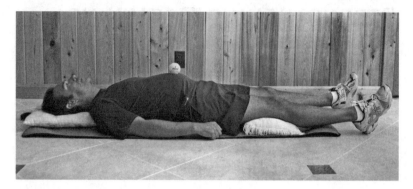

Figure 3.2 Full Breath Exercise, breathing in.

Then gently release air through the mouth and watch the object slowly go down. Breathe out completely, until the object is hidden by your rib cage, as shown in figure 3.3.

Practice taking 10 to 12 full breaths to really feel the process and to memorize the exercise. Then, as you get up and go about your life, try to take a deep breath like this as often as you can. Practice the Full Breath Exercise while standing, sitting, walking, and especially when riding. The more you practice it, the more it becomes engraved in your consciousness and becomes second nature. Repetition will make it become a reflex. Remember, you use your full brain when you take a full breath!

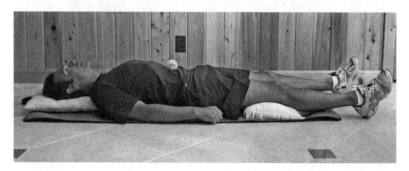

Figure 3.3 Full Breath Exercise, breathing out.

THE DIAPHRAGM BREATHING EXERCISE

Possessing a strong diaphragm muscle is a great advantage in controlling your breathing. The Diaphragm Breathing Exercise is a terrific exercise that will quickly strengthen your diaphragm muscle.

Starting Position

This exercise is best performed while sitting comfortably on a chair, sofa, or bed. Do not lie down. More importantly, do not practice this exercise while standing as you might hyperventilate and risk falling. Being seated will allow you to practice this exercise safely.

Bring your arms up above your head and join your hands together by interlacing your fingers, as shown in figure 3.4.

The Exercise

Gently take a deep full breath through your mouth, stretching your stomach out as shown in figure 3.5. Hold for 2 to 3 seconds before releasing. Every time you take a deep breath, you fully engage your diaphragm muscle.

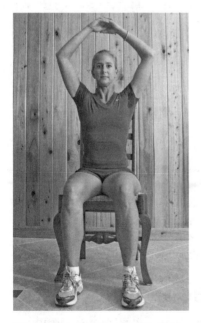
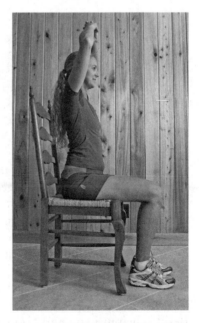

Figure 3.4 Diaphragm Breathing Exercise, starting position.

Figure 3.5 Diaphragm Breathing Exercise, breathing in.

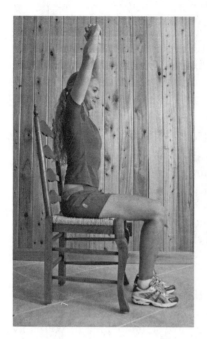

Figure 3.6 Diaphragm Breathing Exercise, breathing out.

After holding your breath for 2 to 3 seconds, breathe out forcefully as if you were blowing out an imaginary candle 10 feet in front of you, as shown in figure 3.6.

Every time you breathe out forcefully, you fully engage your **abdominal** and **intercostal muscles**. Repeat the Diaphragm Breathing Exercise 5 to 10 times in the first week of your exercise regimen. It is normal to feel lightheaded after several diaphragm contractions due to the increased oxygen intake. Simply relax until the sensation disappears. Also, for those of you who are smokers, you might feel your diaphragm muscle cramping the first few times you practice this exercise. When this happens, do not worry. Just relax and practice again a little later. Perseverance will help you release the stress lodged in your diaphragm muscle, and the cramping episodes will disappear as the muscle reclaims its fitness.

By the second week, you should increase your daily practice of this exercise to 12 repetitions. By the third week, you should increase to 20 repetitions. And by the fourth week, you should have no problem completing 30 repetitions without any cramping or feeling lightheaded.

You will feel the benefits of this practice right away. You will be more relaxed and more energized because the oxygen in your system dramatically increases. But most important, daily practice of this exercise will quickly strengthen your diaphragm muscle, giving you more control of your breathing, and creating calmness and composure, which all contribute strongly to a better seat.

BREATHING AND BODY ALIGNMENT

Besides helping you relax and maintain focus, proper breathing plays an important role in helping you align the rib cage over the pelvis. When you take a deep breath, you expand your rib cage and open your chest, helping you bring your shoulders back, and therefore adjusting your overall posture properly over your hips.

Developing a proper breathing technique will enhance your performance not only when riding but in all aspects of your daily life. Full breathing will bring you more vitality in all your activities and relax your mind. Remember, if you use your full lungs, then you use your full brain!

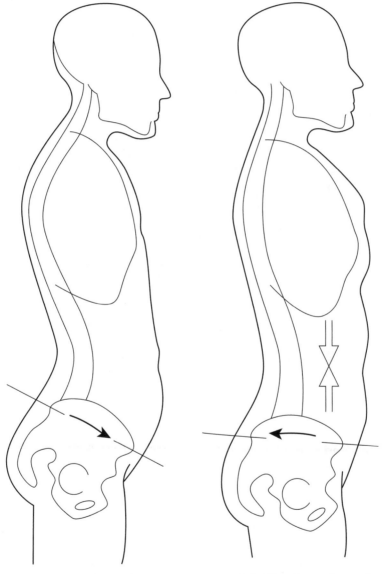

Figure 3.7 This figure shows incorrect body posture. With shallow breathing, the pelvis rolls forward, the chest sinks in, and the arms arch forward, causing a strain on the back shoulder muscles.

Figure 3.8 This figure shows the correct body posture. With proper deep breathing, the pelvis rolls back, the chest lifts, and the arms are properly aligned.

4

Discomfort during riding, or during any activity for that matter, is often linked to the body not being properly aligned. An upright posture is extremely important when riding, so you must learn to develop postural awareness. Having a straight back is not an artificial posture; it is natural to the human body. When you slouch, that is unusual. You cannot breathe properly when you slouch, which often leads to a poor riding performance. Therefore, by sitting properly erect, you maximize your performance toward your optimal seat.

Someone with poor posture typically rides with a rounded upper back, which results in an accentuated forward head posture due to the dropped ribs. A rounded back limits your ability to take a full breath, therefore reducing your relaxation and oxygenation benefits. Furthermore, a rounded back leads to stress buildup in the shoulder muscles, especially the lateral trapezius muscle and the rotator cuff group of muscles (the supraspinatus, the infraspinatus, and the subscapularis muscles). Furthermore, a rounded back creates muscular tightness (or compensation) in the lower back and hips, resulting in poor performance. For a rider, poor posture is a disaster!

To have a straight back, you do not have to strain to pull up your shoulders. The uprightness comes naturally from sitting simply and proudly in your saddle. Because your back is straight, you feel no trace of discomfort or embarrassment, and you develop a good sense of how your head and shoulders should be positioned, too. Then you can allow your legs to brace naturally against the horse's barrel. You complete your posture by holding your hands lightly in front of your navel. This provides a further sense of assuming your proper seat. By remembering the importance of good posture, you are able to synchronize your mind and body.

When your mind and body work together, you never lose your seat.

When your mind and body are unsynchronized, your body will slump. When your body is not properly aligned, you are fighting gravity and your muscles constantly tense up to maintain a sense of balance. Riding like that is very hard work and you will tire quickly.

When your mind and body are synchronized, you achieve good posture because your body is properly aligned and you are breathing naturally. At that point gravity is a benign and positive force that helps you be balanced, be symmetrical in your movements, and enhance your riding seat. Riding in this fashion is much easier.

Any body movement is the harmonious result of the musculoskeletal systems working in unison. The musculoskeletal system is composed of three major systems:

1. The *muscular system*, for power and stabilization;
2. The *fascia system* (a network of connective tissue that surrounds all muscles, bones, and organs throughout the entire body), for support and smoothness; and
3. The *skeletal system* (bones and joints) for support and protection.

When your body is not aligned, your movements become asymmetrical, resulting in a "crooked posture," known in riding as "poor posture." In general, poor posture when sitting, driving, or during certain movement patterns can create physical stress. This physical stress results in stiffness and a limited range of motion. Most people have experienced having one shoulder higher or lower than the other from carrying a heavy bag or briefcase for a long period of time, including the corresponding soreness in the neck and lower back as your whole body adjusted to that imbalance.

Physical trauma also causes the body to compensate in order to protect the injury. Over time, that compensatory movement pattern becomes the "normal" way to move for the body. But your body is still out of alignment, which adversely affects your riding.

This chapter presents two simple self-tests to help you evaluate your overall body alignment. These tests will help you determine your actual body alignment and where you need to focus your efforts right away in order to restore equilibrium and maximize the benefits of the exercises presented later in this book.

First Self-Test:
The Standing Test

This simple test will help you evaluate your actual structural alignment. In classical body alignment evaluation, *proper posture* is
defined by the vertical alignment of the ear, shoulder, hip, knee,
and ankle. In other words, a theoretical plumb line starting at your
ear should pass through the middle of your shoulder, hip, knee,
and ankle as shown in figure 4.1.

Evaluating Your Overall Body
Alignment

Stand in front of a mirror and, with the help of a friend, you can
easily assess your own body alignment. Stand in your usual posture and take a gentle, deep breath. You might want to shift your
weight distribution a little by leaning forward and backward until
you come to the most comfortable position, which is usually
where it takes the least amount of energy to stand up. You just
need to stand relaxed, in bare feet, with your arms by your sides,
looking straight ahead. Have your friend stand behind you and tell
you how your alignment looks. Then make notes on figure 4.2 to
indicate the location and type of alignment problems on your
body.

In gliding sports such as skiing or inline skating, your body
weight should be in front of the heel for optimal performance. If
your body weight falls on the balls of the feet, it means you are
leaning forward a little too much, and that you will quickly strain
your leg extensor muscles (the shin area). If your body weight falls
on the heels of the feet, it means you are leaning back too much.
You risk losing your balance, causing you to tense all your leg and
back flexor muscles (calves), hamstrings, and erector spinae muscles. When standing in front of the mirror and doing a self-test,
ask yourself the following: Do you naturally find your weight
falling in front of your heels? Do you lean slightly forward or
backward?

If the theoretical plumb line starting at your ear falls in front of
your shoulder, hip, knee, and ankle, then you have a lot of "forward head posture." If your shoulders seem to curve strongly
towards your chest, you probably have some degree of *shoulder
kyphosis*, meaning an increased curvature of your spine, which
leads to some degree of rounded shoulders. In order to maintain
a good seat, be sure to control your posture and avoid slouching.

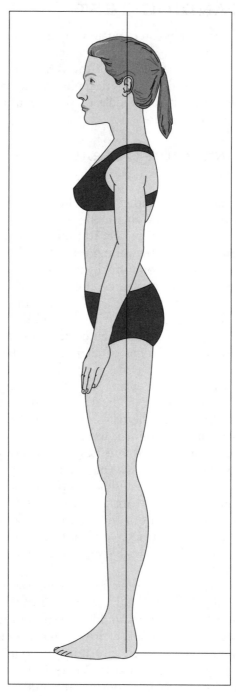

Figure 4.1 Proper body alignment, with theoretical plumb line.

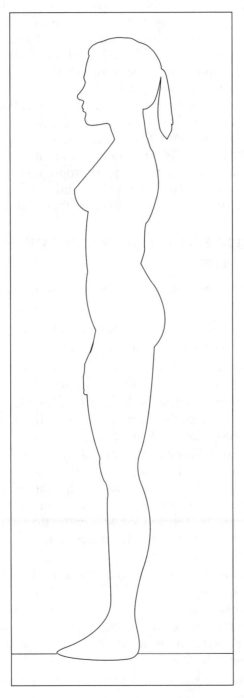

Figure 4.2 Outline of the human body for the standing self-test.

CHECKING YOUR LOWER BACK ALIGNMENT

Another typical rider problem is an excessive lumbar, or lower back, curve. You can easily test your own lower back curve. You just need to stand in a relaxed position against a wall. Make sure your heels, pelvis, upper back, and head are touching the wall. When in this position, try to slide one of your arms in the space between your lower back and the wall. If your arm cannot go through, it means you have a pretty normal curve. If your arm can go through, it means that you have an excessive lumbar curve.

The various exercises offered in this book and specifically the Mid-Back Extension Exercise presented in chapter 9 will work wonders in helping you restore your proper body alignment. As you improve your posture, you will feel more balanced, stronger, and will more likely exercise and ride without suffering injuries.

EVALUATING THE ALIGNMENT OF SPECIFIC BODY PARTS

While standing comfortably in front of a mirror, evaluate the following points:

* **Head.** Is your head straight? Or is it tilted? If tilted, see chapter 9 for shoulder and neck exercises.

* **Chin.** Is your chin sticking out? Or does it lean slightly in? If yes, see chapter 9 for neck exercises.

* **Shoulders.** Look at both shoulders. Are they even? Is one side higher, meaning more contracted? If yes, see chapter 9 for shoulder and neck exercises.

* **Arms and Hands.** Are your arms rotated outward with palms forward? This can reveal tight shoulder muscles. Are your palms facing backward with your elbows sticking slightly out? Even if this is a more natural position, elbows sticking out excessively could indicate tight anterior shoulder and chest muscles. In either case, see chapter 9 for shoulder exercises.

* **Hips.** Are the points of your hips level? If not, see chapter 10 for hip exercises.

* **Legs.** Are your legs aligned? Or are they slightly "bowed"? Or are they *knock-kneed*, meaning they are bent inward? Is one leg rotated outward? If you answer yes to any of these questions, see chapter 10 for leg exercises.

* **Knees.** Are your knees level? If not, see chapter 10 for leg exercises.

❖ **Ankles.** When looking directly down at your feet, can you see your ankles? If yes, that means your chest is well balanced over your hips and that you are in great alignment. If not, adjust your posture by moving your pelvis either forward or backward. If you have to move your pelvis forward, this indicates that there is tension in the back extensor muscles. If you have to move your pelvis backward, then there is tension in your hip flexor muscles. In either case, see chapter 10 for leg and hip exercises.

❖ **Feet.** Do your feet open outward? This means tension is in your gluteus muscle. Do your feet close in? If so, then tension is in your adductor muscles and internal rotator muscles. Are your feet standing awkwardly? This is indicative of open hips and probably of lower abdominal muscle tension. See chapter 10 for leg exercises that will also help with your feet.

❖ **Arches.** Is your body weight falling over your inner or outer arch? Either one is a sign of an imbalance between the flexor, extensor, and adductor muscle groups of your leg. A quick look at the soles of your shoes or riding boots will be revealing. Are they worn out on the inner or outer arch? If not, then your weight is properly balanced between both arches. If they show wear, see chapter 10 for leg exercises that will also help with your arches.

SECOND SELF-TEST: THE WALKING TEST

This second test will help you evaluate your body's alignment while you are in motion.

Casually walk in a straight line as you take a gentle, but deep breath. As you walk, observe the points listed below and make notes on figure 4.3 to indicate the location of alignment problems on your body.

❖ **Legs.** How far do your legs reach with each stride? Are they even in their stride?

❖ **Back.** How does your lower back feel? Do you feel stiffer on one side?

❖ **Shoulders.** How are your shoulders moving around your spinal axis?

❖ **Arms.** Are your arms moving evenly? Is one side stiffer than the other?

❖ **Neck.** Does your neck lean forward or is your chin placed slightly back?

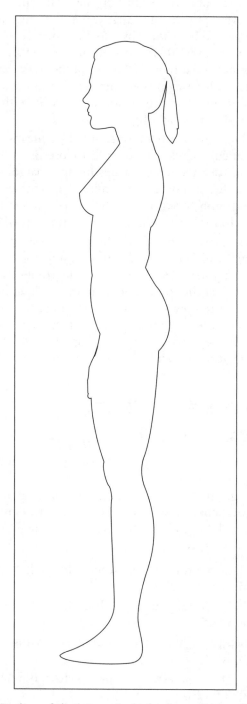

Figure 4.3 Outline of the human body for the walking self-test.

Observing your body during the walking test will give you more information about your overall balance. To correct the various imbalances noticed when walking, please see the section "Evaluating the Alignment of Specific Body Parts" and refer to the corresponding exercise for each imbalance.

Tips to improve your postural alignment: As you walk, try to feel your legs starting from your rib cage instead of your hips. This will engage your core muscles and give you better stability. Also, as your heel hits the ground, feel your weight moving forward across the foot to the middle of the ball of the foot. It will help balance the leg muscles.

5

Understanding the benefits of stretching and how to properly stretch will maximize the results of your exercise program. Having a thorough knowledge of the correct way to stretch each body part will help you evaluate your body regularly and choose the appropriate exercise to increase your fitness. A regular stretching program prevents muscle problems, provides relaxation, and develops body awareness.

Important Note: If you had any recent physical problems such as a fall, a direct trauma, or surgery, particularly of the joints and muscles, please consult your doctor before you start a stretching program.

BENEFITS OF REGULAR STRETCHING

Stretching improves your coordination and allows you to evaluate your actual physical condition. Regular stretching exercises provide both physical and cerebral benefits.

Keep in mind that, due to similar physiological properties, the same benefits of stretching apply to your horse. This is why it is important that you take the time to stretch your horse's legs, back, and neck. For more information on how to properly stretch a horse, consult the author's *Equine Massage: A Practical Guide, Second Edition* (John Wiley & Sons, 2007).

PHYSICAL BENEFITS

The musculoskeletal benefits of frequent stretching exercises include increased flexibility, prevention of injuries, improved general metabolism, and better movement.

Flexibility—Stretching keeps muscle fibers and joints flexible. When you stretch a muscle, you lengthen its fibers. This action mechanically affects the sensory nerve cells and resets the feedback mechanism to the central nervous system. The result is a widening of the blood vessels, improved tone of the muscle fibers, and increased elasticity of the ligaments and the joint capsules, which allows for freer, easier, more controlled, and quicker movements— all resulting in better overall coordination in your seat.

Prevention of injuries—Stretching reduces muscle tension and therefore helps to prevent muscle pulls. In addition, it also loosens the ligaments and joint capsules and makes the body feel more relaxed. It releases muscle contractures due to old scar tissue, helps to relieve muscle pain from chronic tension, and reduces post-exercise soreness and stiffness.

Metabolism—Muscle stretching increases blood and lymph circulation, bringing more oxygen and nutrients to body parts. Stretching also helps prevent inflammation and adhesion formation (scar tissue), trigger points, and stress point buildup.

Movement—Regular stretching will improve the range of motion of your joints, contribute to loosening your various layers of fascia, and improve your overall coordination and the response time of your reflexes.

You will feel the physiological benefits of regular stretching exercises immediately, and a daily routine will provide the most benefit. You should practice some stretching exercises just before riding as a warm-up.

CEREBRAL BENEFITS

Cerebral refers to the nervous system control center—the brain, the spinal cord, and the nerve plexus. A person's "body awareness" is, of course, cerebral (mental). Hence, one part of stretching is cerebral because the activity develops body awareness. Stretching various body parts helps you to focus on them and to become in touch with them mentally. This process develops your self-awareness, thereby improving your coordination in all aspects of movement.

The stretching of muscles sends relaxation impulses—via the sensory neuron—to the central nervous system, reflexively loosening your mind's control over your body. Stretching also decreases motor neuron tension transmitted throughout the body. You will relax both physically and mentally, which are important factors when dealing with stress. Stretching will indirectly help you to release subconscious anxiety associated with muscle tension.

Stretching also gives you feedback on the health of the muscle groups and the ligaments, particularly in regard to their elasticity and tone.

When to Stretch

Muscles, tendons, and ligaments (and eventually joint capsules) may become damaged if they are stretched when cold. Stretching after a short warm-up period, such as a walk, will limit the risk of injury that results from overstretching. It is best to stretch as a cool-down immediately after training.

That said, you can stretch at any time. Stretching should be done every day, after every training or riding session. A regular routine will give you feedback on your physical condition, including the flexibility of your joints, the agility of your muscle groups, and the progression of your training program.

The Stretch Reflex

The *stretch reflex* is a protective mechanism that prevents a muscle from being overstretched and torn. The stretch reflex is a nervous reaction caused when the muscle spindle, a sensory nerve cell, is overstretched. When overstretched, the muscle spindle fires nerve impulses to the spinal cord. The reflex arc mechanism (located in the spine) then fires back motor neuron impulses that cause an instant muscle contraction. This contraction prevents the muscle from being injured. So do not overstretch and do not try to reach beyond the muscle's maximum flexibility. Instead, just hold the stretch in a relaxed manner and for a longer period of time. Your flexibility will increase naturally when you start stretching regularly.

What to Stretch

Throughout all three programs offered in this book, you will be stretching these aspects of your body: your back, neck, shoulders, and legs. After exercising each body part, you will immediately stretch it in order to maintain suppleness and prevent stiffness. Regardless of the part being stretched, observe the following important guidelines in order to maximize your stretching benefits.

How to Stretch

To obtain the best results, you need to respect the structures you are stretching. To stretch correctly, it is important to be concerned with your natural body alignment. Always move and stretch your limbs in their natural range of motion. Do not do abnormal twists or torque parts of your body. When starting your stretching routine, it is very important to focus on quality of movement rather than speed of execution.

Important Note: Stretching is not a contest to see how far you can stretch or to go further each time you do it. The object of stretching is to relax muscle and ligament tension in order to promote freer movement and to trigger the other benefits listed earlier. To achieve all of this, you need to stretch safely, starting with the easy stretch described later in this chapter and building to a regular, deeper stretch. Never go too far; the stretch reflex will cause the muscle to contract to prevent tearing of the fibers.

Stretching should always be done in a relaxed and steady manner. The first time you stretch, do it slowly and gently. Give yourself time to adjust your body and mind to the physical and mental stress release that stretching initiates. The stretch should be tailored to your particular muscular structure, flexibility, and level of tension. Again, to avoid the risk of tearing your muscle and/or ligament fibers, do not overstretch.

Do not let your mind wander when stretching. Take gentle deep breaths to help you stay focused and relaxed. This approach will heighten your perceptions and give you a more refined touch. Staying calm will allow you to better feel your body not only during stretching exercises but also when riding. You will be amazed by the sensations generated by this practice.

When you engage in stretching a body part, start with the easy stretch for 10 to 15 seconds, and then follow with the deeper stretch for a few additional seconds to get the most out of your performance.

THE EASY STRETCH

Always begin your stretching routine with the easy stretch. Stretch only about 80 percent of the total stretching capability of that particular body part and hold it for 10 to 15 seconds (two full deep breaths). You will enjoy this gentle approach. Be steady when performing this stretch. Never move hastily or jerkily. Do not pull excessively on any body part because you risk tearing muscle fibers by overstretching.

THE DEEPER STRETCH

Once you get used to the easy stretch, you can work into the deeper stretch. After the initial 10 seconds of the easy stretch and as your muscle tightness decreases, adjust your grip until you again feel some tension. Hold for another 5 seconds. Repeat two to three times until you feel you have reached the maximum stretching capacity of the muscle. Avoid triggering the stretch reflex by overstretching. Be in control, breathing calmly.

Always start with the easy stretch for 10 to 15 seconds (a couple of deep breaths), then work into the deeper stretch. This activity will finely tune your muscles and increase your overall flexibility. Do not make jerky or bouncy movements. Never stretch an *acutely* (recently) torn muscle. Never force the joint into any abnormal range or twist it. Always stretch the *agonist muscle* (the one responsible for the action) and its *antagonist muscle* (the one that has to let go for the action to happen). A regular practice of stretching with comfortable and painless movements will help you go beyond your current flexibility limit and allow you to come closer to your full potential.

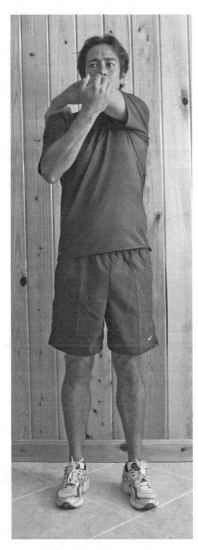 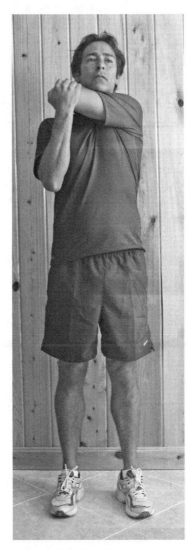

Figure 5.1 The easy stretch of the left triceps muscle.

Figure 5.2 The deeper stretch of the left triceps muscle.

MENTALLY COUNTING A STRETCH

The time frame in which you stretch a muscle is very important. At first, silently count the seconds for each stretch. This will ensure that you hold its tension for the correct length of time. After a while, you will develop a feel for this practice and will subconsciously know when you have reached your full stretching capability without having to count. This practice of mental counting will help you get the best results from the stretching technique.

Another approach to counting is to take deep breaths. Instead of counting the seconds and being impatient, you can take deep breaths. For the average person, the "in" and "out" of a full, relaxed, and deep breath takes about 7 to 8 seconds. So, just concentrate on taking 2 to 3 deep breaths while holding your stretch. This practice of deep breathing will relax you and maximize your stretching benefits.

OVERALL BENEFITS OF STRETCHING

Regular stretching will improve the range of motion of the joints, your overall coordination, and the response time of your reflexes, not to mention your overall relaxation. The physiological benefits of stretching exercises upon the body are immediate.

6

EXERCISE TIPS
AND SUGGESTIONS

This chapter explains the benefits of exercising and how to properly exercise in order to maximize your benefits. When exercising, it is important to maintain balance between the various muscle groups. In conventional workouts, strong muscles tend to get stronger and weak muscles tend to get weaker, resulting in muscular imbalance, a primary cause of injury and chronic back pain.

The exercise programs presented in chapters 12 through 14 will help you work better from your core, which in turn strengthens your back, neck, legs, and arms, and improves your strength and coordination while minimizing the risk of injury. These exercises are especially beneficial to riders, who commonly experience back injuries from riding. An added bonus is that these exercises can be performed in your home, so you don't have to spend money on gym fees. It is a great feeling to be able to exercise in the convenience of your home and see quick results.

Important Note: If you had any recent heart problems, or other physical problems, please consult your doctor before you start this exercise program.

BENEFITS OF REGULAR EXERCISE

Exercising regularly improves your muscle tone and develops strength, agility, and economy of motion resulting in better movement and a reduction of musculoskeletal injury. Regular exercise increases circulation, improves general metabolism, and tends to improve your mood, too.

Muscle tone—When exercising, you contract and relax the muscles so many times that it results in a slight widening of the blood vessels and muscle fibers become more toned.

Muscle strength—The repetition of the exercises will cause the body to develop more muscle fibers, resulting in stronger muscles.

Muscle agility—With stronger muscles you will be able to better control the amount of contraction desired between agonist and antagonist muscles during any movement, resulting in finesse and agility of execution.

Prevention of injuries—Exercising helps maintain a stronger muscle tone throughout the body. This in turn provides better support to joints, thereby preventing ligament and joint capsule sprains during jolting movements. Also, stronger muscles have more endurance, cutting down the risk of inflammation when riding long hours.

Metabolism—When exercising, the repetition of the muscle contraction-relaxation cycle has a pumping effect on both the blood and lymph circulation. This results in more oxygen and nutrients flowing to the body parts and toxins being more efficiently evacuated.

Improvements—Regular exercise improves the tone and strength of your muscle groups, resulting in better control and coordination.

The physiological benefits of regular exercise upon the body are immediate. So you should definitely include these exercises in your preparation for riding. Exercising 2 to 3 times a week will secure all of the above benefits; however, a daily routine will benefit you the most.

WHEN TO EXERCISE

The morning is the best time of day to perform your exercise routine because it gets your body ready for the day. However, exercising during the day or evening is fine. Regardless of your schedule preference, you should always start with a few minutes of cardiovascular activity (see chapter 7) to warm up your body and to get it ready for more exercises. Maintaining a daily schedule of exercise will maximize all the benefits listed above and quickly get you to your best physical condition.

HOW TO EXERCISE

To attain the best results, it is important to be concerned with your natural body alignment. When starting out, focusing on the quality of movement rather than the quantity is important. In due time, you will gradually build up to a greater number of repetitions.

You should use the results of the self-testing exercises presented in chapter 4 as a starting point for your exercise program. Each exercise presented in this book is described step-by-step to give you maximum guidance. Follow the guidelines for the proper positioning and development of the exercise, for the suggested number of repetitions, and for the mode of breathing.

While exercising, use your full range of motion. A muscle that goes through its full range of motion mobilizes more muscle fibers, which helps to develop stronger muscles.

Important Note: Exercising is not a contest to see how strong you are. Do not force an exercise because you run the risk of injuring your muscles or ligaments. The object of exercising is to develop your muscle tone, balance, and agility in order for you to acquire a better seat.

Exercising should always be done in a relaxed and steady manner. Work out slowly and gently. Give yourself time to feel the burn in your muscles throughout the entire exercise. Breathe slowly and deeply. You should exhale during the contraction of your muscles and inhale when relaxing the muscles.

STAYING FOCUSED WHEN YOU EXERCISE

As mentioned earlier, when exercising, do not let your mind wander. By practicing deep breathing, you will stay focused, yet relaxed, which will enhance your perceptions and effectiveness. This sense of calm will allow you to better evaluate the work your muscles are going through during exercises and also when riding.

PHYSICAL BENEFITS OF EXERCISE

Regular exercise will improve your muscle tone and stamina. In turn, it will give you better control over your seat and movements, and give you more power and agility, resulting in greater finesse of execution while riding.

7

WARM-UP EXERCISES

Warming up your body prior to exercise is very important. It loosens your muscles, increases your circulation, gets you ready for your exercises, and reduces the risk of injuring your body. The best way to warm up your body is to spend a few minutes doing some cardiovascular activity. You will get results so much faster when you include cardiovascular exercises in your fitness-training program. This chapter covers some simple cardiovascular exercises that you can easily perform for a few minutes prior to your exercise routine. No equipment is required. You will use these warm-up exercises in the beginning, intermediate, and advanced exercise programs presented in chapters 12 through 14.

Important Note: If you have a serious heart condition, you should consult your doctor first before performing the following exercises.

WALKING ON THE SPOT EXERCISE

The Walking on the Spot Exercise is one of the most efficient cardiovascular exercises you can do. Go easy at the beginning. You will quickly see that this exercise gives you a "run for your money."

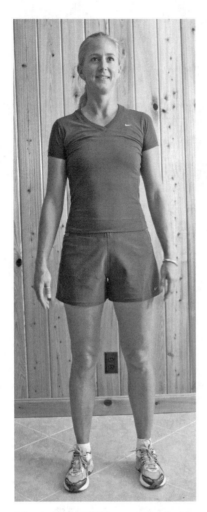

Figure 7.1 Walking on the Spot Exercise, starting position.

STARTING POSITION

Stand relaxed, away from any object or furniture. You can keep your arms at your sides or you can bend your elbows if you wish.

THE EXERCISE

Start the exercise by gently bringing your left knee up toward your left chest, as shown in figure 7.2, and slowly release back to your starting position. Then bring your right knee toward your right chest as shown in figure 7.3 and slowly release back to the starting position.

Take your time during this exercise as it will stretch your gluteals and hamstrings and get you ready for the next phase. Repeat 3 times, alternating each side.

Next, keep walking on the spot; however, you only need to raise your knee high enough for your thigh to be at a 90-degree angle to your body, as shown in figures 7.4 and 7.5. Remember to alternate legs.

Important Note: As you raise your knees, instead of pulling from the hip point, imagine that you are pulling from your rib cage. By exercising in this manner, you will engage your abdominal muscles more efficiently, contributing to the development of your core muscles.

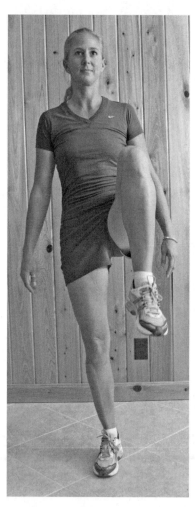

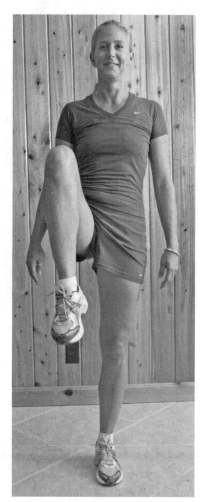

Figure 7.2 Walking on the Spot Exercise, left leg.

Figure 7.3 Walking on the Spot Exercise, right leg.

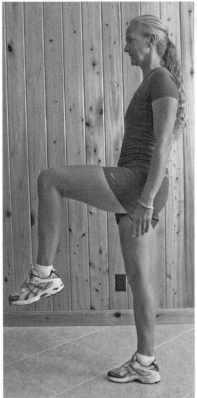 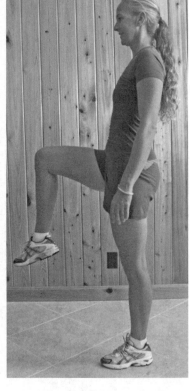

Figure 7.4 Walking on the Spot Exercise, left leg at 90 degrees.   *Figure 7.5 Walking on the Spot Exercise, right leg at 90 degrees.*

At the beginning of your practice, repeat this warm-up exercise 20 to 30 times. By the second week, you should build up to 50 repetitions. In the early aspects of your practice, your pace should be to lift a leg every 3 seconds. As you improve your stamina and coordination, you can speed up your rhythm by lifting your leg every 2 seconds or less.

ADVANCED VERSION OF WALKING ON THE SPOT EXERCISE

When you begin the intermediate exercise program, please consider adding this new level of difficulty to the Walking on the Spot Exercise. Take a few steps in which you bring each knee all the way up to the *opposite* side of your chest. Bring your left knee to your right chest as shown in figure 7.6. Then lift your right knee to the left chest as shown in figure 7.7.

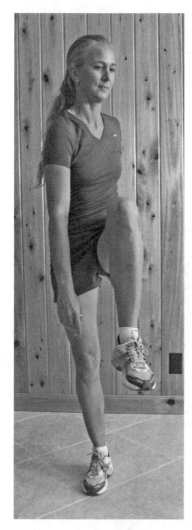 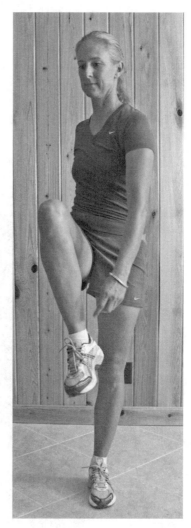

Figure 7.6 Advanced Walking
on the Spot Exercise, left
knee up to right chest.

Figure 7.7 Advanced Walking
on the Spot Exercise, right
knee up to left chest.

This advanced version of the Walking on the Spot Exercise will really get you going. A 2- to 3-minute interval is plenty of time to sufficiently warm up before you start exercising. However, if you wish to perform this exercise for 5 minutes or more, it will strengthen your heart. Start slowly and build up as you see fit.

SCISSOR FEET EXERCISE

The Scissor Feet Exercise is a very efficient cardiovascular warm-up exercise. However, if your knees give you grief, take it easy at first to see if this exercise is right for you.

STARTING POSITION

To begin the exercise, stand relaxed with your feet shoulder width apart, as shown in figure 7.8.

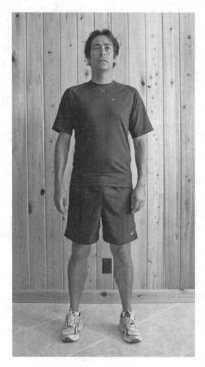

Figure 7.8 Scissor Feet Exercise,
starting position.

THE EXERCISE

In a quick step, move your left foot forward and your right foot backward at the same time, as shown in figure 7.9.

Then, in another quick step, bring your feet back to the starting position as shown in figure 7.8. Repeat the quick step, but this time bring your right foot forward and your left foot backward, as shown in figure 7.10.

Then move back to the starting position, as shown in figure 7.8.

This pattern creates a scissor motion between your feet. Repeat the exercise 10 to 15 times in the beginning, increasing to 25 repetitions when comfortable.

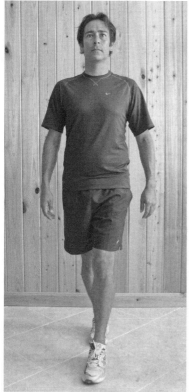

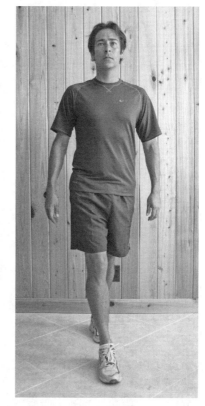

Figure 7.9 Scissor Feet Exercise, left front.

Figure 7.10 Scissor Feet Exercise, left behind.

ARM TWIST EXERCISE

The Arm Twist Exercise is a good cardiovascular exercise because it involves your abdominal wall muscles.

STARTING POSITION

Before you start this exercise, stand relaxed with your feet shoulder-width apart, and bend your arms at the elbow. Then lift your arms to shoulder height, as shown in figure 7.11.

You can extend or flex your forearm if you like; however, keep your elbow at shoulder height during the entire exercise.

THE EXERCISE

Start the exercise by loosening your waistline. To do so, rotate your upper body to the left so you are turning 90 degrees from your starting position, as shown in figure 7.12.

Figure 7.11 Arm Twist Exercise, starting position.

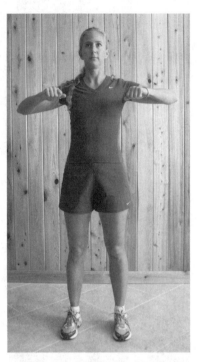

Next, return to your starting position and then turn your upper body to the right so you are turning 90 degrees from the starting position, as shown in figure 7.13.

You can repeat this exercise slowly 6 more times on each side to really loosen your hips, lower back, and abdominal muscles.

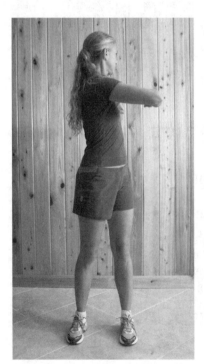

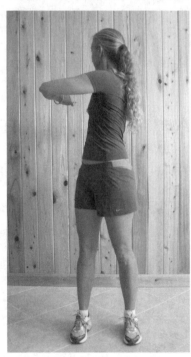

Figure 7.12 Arm Twist Exercise, turning left.

Figure 7.13 Arm Twist Exercise, turning right.

ADVANCED VERSION OF
ARM TWIST EXERCISE

You can continue the Arm Twist Exercise by doing an advanced version, in which you slightly increase the pace and lift your knees. So when you rotate to the left, lift the left knee up and toward the right shoulder as shown in figure 7.14.

Next, rotate to the right and lift your right knee up and toward the left shoulder, as shown in figure 7.15.

Repeat the advanced version of the Arm Twist Exercise 5 to 10 times in the beginning, gradually building up to 20 repetitions.

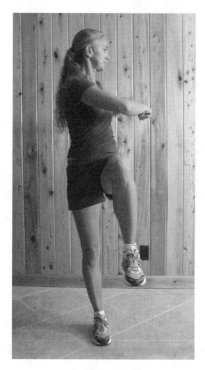
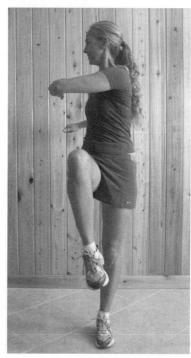

Figure 7.14 Advanced Arm Twist Exercise, turning left and lifting left knee to right shoulder.

Figure 7.15 Advanced Arm Twist Exercise, turning right and lifting right knee to left shoulder.

Conclusion

The exercises presented in this chapter will give you great cardio-vascular warm-up benefits in a short time, 2 to 5 minutes before you begin exercising. However, if you wish to develop a strong heart and endurance capabilities, you should consider practicing an aerobic activity 2 to 3 times a week, for 30 to 45 minutes at a time. You can choose from a variety of exercises such as walking, jogging, cycling, climbing up and down sets of stairs, jumping rope, using a stepping machine, running or walking on a treadmill, and so on. Alternating between these various exercise options prevents boredom and contributes to your overall cross-training fitness.

8

CORE MUSCLE EXERCISES AND STRETCHES

Possessing a strong core is crucial in any athletic performance. For riders, the weakest and most injured area is the lower back. Why is that? During riding, the lower back and hip area are the stable portions of the body. In order to stay balanced on the horse, the core muscles constantly act as stabilizers, receiving a lot of pull from both the upper and the lower body. If your abdominal muscles, which are part of your core muscles, are not strong, the back muscles carry all of the stabilizing effort, which increases the risk of soreness and injury in that area.

Proper use of the abdominal wall is essential in developing a strong core. During any exercise, as you contract your abdominal muscles and bring your navel in, the abdominal wall stabilizes the spine—the inner abdominals stabilize the spinal column while the outer abdominals provide general stabilization and assist with motion.

To feel your deepest abdominal muscle, the transversus abdominis, start by lying on your back and relaxing. When ready, cough once. The muscle you feel contracting is your transversus abdominis. Repeat the coughing several times, and then hold your transversus abdominis contracted for a few seconds. This exercise helps you to become acquainted with this muscle. Later it will be easier for you to contract your entire core muscle group when riding.

If you are not strong and flexible in the core area of your body, you will get injured. It is as simple as that. A strong core is essential for good posture and athletic performance, and contributes to a healthy and good-looking body.

The following muscles are considered core muscles:

1. The abdominal muscle group

- *External oblique* (runs along the sides and front of the abdomen and is used for downward pull)
- *Internal oblique* (lies under the external oblique muscle and is used for upward pull)
- *Transversus abdominis* (innermost abdominal muscle that runs horizontally and is underneath the internal oblique muscle)
- *Rectus abdominis* (vertical-running front muscle; called a *six-pack* if well-defined)

2. The stabilizer muscles of the spine, which include the back (erector spinae) group of muscles

- *Iliocostalis* (cervicis, lumborum, and thoracis sections)
- *Longissimus* (capitis, cervicis, and thoracis sections)
- *Spinalis* (capitis, cervicis, and thoracis sections)

For more detailed information about the core muscles, see chapter 2 and figures 2.6 and 2.7.

To smoothly develop and strengthen your core muscles, specifically the abdominals and back (erector spinae) muscles, you should perform the following simple exercises that will bring you quick results. Also, two great stretches are provided to help you maintain the flexibility of these core muscles. Because you will be warming up your body before exercising (see chapter 7), there is no need to stretch before your workout. Stretching is most beneficial to perform after exercising. However, this is not carved in stone. If you wish to stretch before performing each strengthening exercise, please feel free to do so. But make sure you stretch afterward, too.

Strengthening Exercises for the Core Muscles

Abdominal Muscles Exercise

The Abdominal Muscles Exercise engages all your abdominal muscles at one time. Except for your anterior neck muscles, no other muscles are used during this exercise so you get a real "abs workout" to quickly develop and strengthen these muscles. Another great benefit of this particular exercise is that it will help flatten your stomach!

Starting Position

Lie comfortably on your back, with your knees bent and the palms of your hands resting on your chest, as shown in figure 8.1. You might want to place a soft pillow underneath your lower back and/or neck for comfort. Raise your head and shoulders off the floor, using only your abdominal muscles.

Before you start the crunch, make sure that you gently push your lower back (*sacrum*) against the floor and that your shoulders are lying flat against the floor. This will prevent you from using your hip flexor and pectoral muscles. And remember to only use your abdominal muscles to raise your head and shoulders.

The Exercise

Start the exercise by taking a deep breath. As you slowly exhale, bring your chin towards your chest, as shown in figure 8.2.

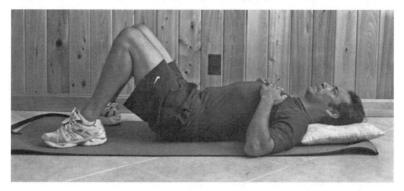

Figure 8.1 Abdominal Muscles Exercise, starting position.

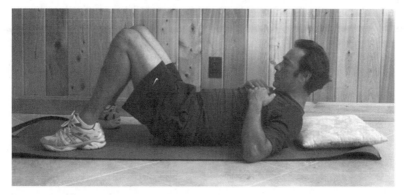

Figure 8.2 Abdominal Muscles Exercise, "chin in" position.

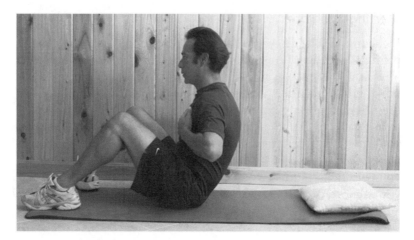

Figure 8.3 Abdominal Muscles Exercise, ending position.

Then lift your chest off the ground, rolling toward your knees. Keep your buttocks against the floor and your hands on your chest with your shoulders drawn back, as shown in figure 8.3.

With practice you should be able to perform this entire movement in one long motion during your complete exhalation. When you reach your knees, hold 2 seconds. Then, gently and slowly, let yourself roll back as you inhale again. This exercise activates all the abdominal muscles. Do not go too fast; stay in control. Feel all aspects of your abdominal muscles as they are exercised. Repeat 6 times in the very beginning of your exercise program, building up toward 12 repetitions in one session by the end of your intermediate program.

ADVANCED VERSION OF ABDOMINAL MUSCLES EXERCISE

An advanced variation of the Abdominal Muscles Exercise will strengthen the transversus abdominis and oblique muscles on the sides of the abdominal wall. But this time as you perform the crunch, instead of bringing yourself straight up and dead center with your knees (as you did previously), pull yourself up and toward the left knee, as shown in figure 8.4.

Repeat by pulling yourself up and toward the right knee, as shown in figure 8.5.

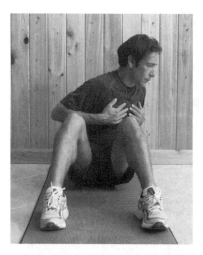 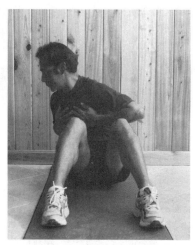

Figure 8.4 Advanced Abdominal
Muscles Exercise, bringing
chest to left knee, legs at a
90-degree angle.

Figure 8.5 Advanced Abdominal
Muscles Exercise, bringing
chest to right knee, legs at a
90-degree angle.

BACK MUSCLES EXERCISE

This exercise develops and strengthens your back muscles. A strong back will benefit your spinal structure because it is important to maintain a balance of muscle power between your back and your core muscles.

Starting Position

Position yourself comfortably on your stomach, with legs straight and your arms extended above your head, as shown in figure 8.6. You might want to place a soft pillow underneath your belly or face for comfort.

The Exercise

Start the exercise by taking a deep breath. As you slowly exhale, simultaneously lift your legs, head, chest, and arms, keeping your arms straight out, as shown in figure 8.7.

Raise your arms and leg as much as you can off the floor! When you have reached your maximum extension, hold for 2 seconds. Then relax, returning slowly to your original position as you inhale again. Do not go too fast; stay in control. Feel all aspects of your back muscles as they get exercised. Repeat 5 to 6 times in the beginning exercise program, building up toward 12 repetitions in one session by the end of the intermediate exercise program.

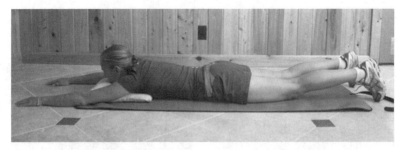

Figure 8.6 Back Muscles Exercise, starting position.

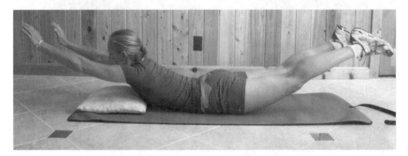

Figure 8.7 Back Muscles Exercise, ending position.

STRETCHES FOR THE CORE MUSCLES

ABDOMINAL MUSCLES STRETCH

Starting Position

Lie down comfortably on your stomach with your legs straight, toes pointing perpendicular to the floor. Place your hands by the sides of your chest, with elbows bent, as shown in figure 8.8.

The Stretch

Start this exercise by taking a deep breath. Then, as you slowly exhale, lift your head, shoulders, and chest up while you keep the lower body on the floor. Use your hands and arms to assist your extension until the end of the easy stretch, meaning when you feel the points of your hips start to lift away from the floor. However, your hip points should stay in contact with the floor at all times, as shown in figure 8.9.

Next, once you reach your full extension, take three gentle full breaths while you feel the stretch in your abdominal wall, which

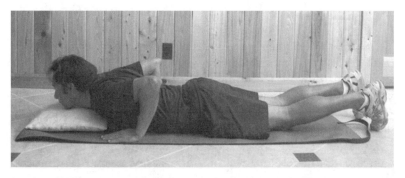

Figure 8.8 Abdominal Muscles Stretch, starting position.

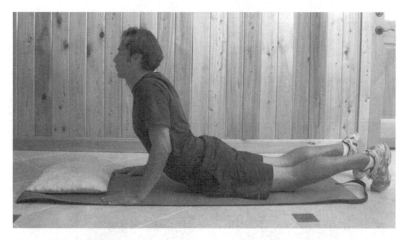

Figure 8.9 Abdominal Muscles Stretch, ending position.

is about 10 seconds. Try to arch your back some more for a deeper stretch. However, do not overarch your back. Stop the stretch if you feel any discomfort in your back. Keep your hip points in contact with the floor. Hold for another few breaths.

Then slowly lower your body back to your starting position during an exhalation.

BACK MUSCLES STRETCH

Starting Position

The Back Muscles Stretch is best done while sitting in a chair in an upright position. Place your legs so your knees are shoulder-width apart, as shown in figure 8.10.

The Stretch

To begin this exercise, take a deep breath. Then as you slowly exhale, curl your body forward while you slowly tighten your abdominal muscles. Continue until your shoulders rest on your knees, as shown in figure 8.11.

Maintain this position, relaxing in the easy stretch with three slow full breaths.

For a deeper stretch, gently tuck your chin in until it touches your breastbone. Hold this position for a few more deep breaths. When done, release your chin and while exhaling slowly return to your starting position.

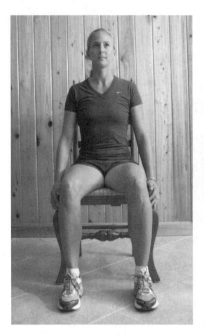

Figure 8.10 Back Muscles Stretch, starting position.

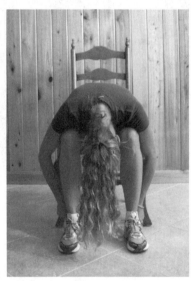

Figure 8.11 Back Muscles Stretch, ending position.

9

UPPER BODY EXERCISES AND STRETCHES

Possessing a strong upper body is important in riding because it helps you with your balance and overall riding style. In order to stay with your horse's center of gravity, you must constantly align your upper body with your core muscles while easily and delicately maneuvering the reins. Tension in your upper body leads to neck and shoulder stiffness and eventually to soreness.

By upper body, I mean the neck, shoulders, and upper torso. (See figures 2.3 and 2.4 in chapter 2 for illustrations of the muscles.) The following muscles are considered the upper body:

Neck Muscles

- The levator scapulae muscles
- The scalene muscles

Shoulder Muscles

- The deltoid muscles (anterior, middle, and posterior)
- The rotator cuff muscles (supraspinatus, infraspinatus, and subscapularis)
- The teres muscles (minor and major)
- The trapezius muscles (upper and lower)

Upper Torso Muscles

- The coracobrachialis muscles
- The latissimus dorsi muscles
- The longissimus muscles (capitis, cervicis, and thoracis)
- The pectoralis muscles (minor and major)
- The rhomboid muscles (minor and major)
- The spinalis muscles (capitis, cervicis, and thoracis)

The neck performs flexion (flexing movement), extension, and side movements. The shoulders perform *abduction* (moving away from the body), *adduction* (pulling toward the body), sideward elevation, and *circumduction* (circular movements of a limb). In order to keep a good seat, your upper body, like your core, needs to be strong. A strong upper body contributes to good posture, agility, athletic performance, and finesse of execution.

Next are some simple exercises that will safely develop the muscles of your upper body. Regular practice of these exercises will strengthen these muscles, which need to be strong for good riding. Before starting, warm up with some exercises presented in chapter 7 to increase your blood circulation and prepare your muscles for their workout. Afterwards, follow the stretching recommendations to help loosen your muscles, maintain their maximum flexibility, and prevent stiffness.

Strengthening Exercises for the Upper Body

Neck Exercises

For a good posture, proper use of the neck is essential. In order to keep your entire spine properly aligned during exercise, tuck your chin slightly in. This technique, combined with the correct use of your core muscles, greatly helps you secure a good seat during any motion. The following exercises will strengthen your neck so that you will naturally hold your head more erect, contributing to an elegant riding style.

Neck Flexion Exercise

This exercise strengthens your neck flexor muscles, which better enables you to stabilize the movement of your head, especially during the posting trot.

Starting Position
Sit comfortably on a chair and place the palms of both hands over your forehead, as shown in figure 9.1.

The Exercise
Start the exercise by taking a deep breath. As you slowly exhale, tuck your chin as close as possible to your neck and chest and simultaneously resist the motion with your hands, as shown in figure 9.2. Maintain your contraction through the

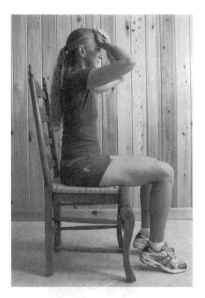
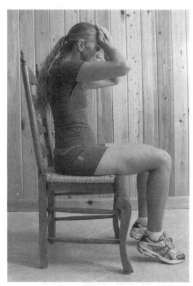

*Figure 9.1 Neck Flexion
Exercise, starting position.*

*Figure 9.2 Neck Flexion
Exercise, ending position.*

entire exhalation. Push as hard as you wish without creating any discomfort.

When you are done with the contraction, relax your hands and slowly roll your neck back to an upward position as you inhale again. Repeat 3 to 5 times in the early aspects of your exercise regimen, building up to 10 repetitions in one session by the end of your beginning program. You can also increase the intensity of the exercise by increasing the resistance created by your hands.

Neck Extension Exercise

This exercise strengthens your neck extensor muscles, which enable you to stabilize the movement of your head, especially during the posting trot.

Starting Position
Sitting comfortably in a chair, place the palms of both your hands on the back of your head, as shown in figure 9.3.

The Exercise
Start the exercise by taking a deep breath. As you slowly exhale, extend your neck backward, but gently resist the motion with your hands, as shown in figure 9.4. Maintain your contraction through the entire breath.

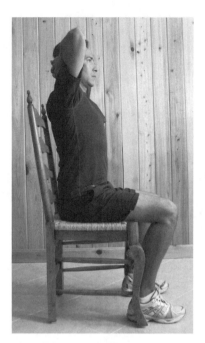 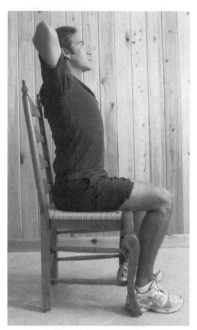

Figure 9.3 Neck Extension
Exercise, starting position.

Figure 9.4 Neck Extension
Exercise, ending position.

When you are done, relax your neck and hands, and as you inhale again, gently bring your neck back into a forward position. Repeat 3 to 5 times in the early aspect of your exercise regimen, building up to 10 repetitions in one session by the end of your beginning program. You can also increase the intensity of the exercise by increasing the resistance created by your hands.

Advanced Version of the Neck Extension Exercise

If you found your head posture was too forward when you performed the overall posture self-test, you should practice this more efficient, advanced version of the Neck Extension Exercise. This exercise quickly helps you to develop stronger neck and upper back muscles as well as addresses your head posture.

Starting Position

Lie comfortably on your back with your knees bent and a rolled towel under the back of your neck. The rolled towel should be

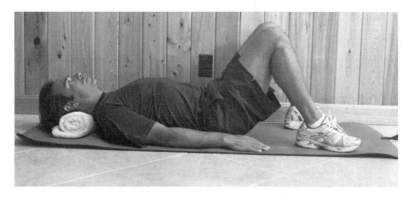

Figure 9.5 Advanced Neck Extension Exercise, starting position.

about 2 to 3 inches in diameter to best fit your neck, as shown in figure 9.5.

The Exercise
Take a deep breath to start the exercise. As you slowly exhale, push your neck backward against the floor (and against the towel) by contracting your back muscles. Maintain your contraction through the entire breath, as shown in figure 9.6.

When you are done, relax your muscles and gently bring your chin slightly in as you inhale again. Repeat the exercise 3 to 5 times in the early aspect of your exercise regimen, building up to 10 repetitions in one session by the end of your beginning exercise program.

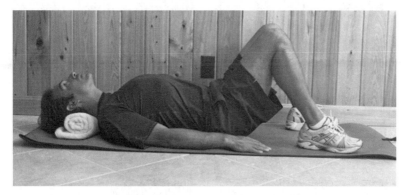

Figure 9.6 Advanced Neck Extension Exercise, ending position.

Neck Half Rolls Exercise

The Neck Half Rolls Exercise will help you to alternately contract each side of the neck while stretching the opposite side. Several daily repetitions will strengthen these muscles, providing better support and control of your neck movements.

Starting Position
Sitting comfortably on a chair, let your arms hang loosely by the sides of your body as shown in figure 9.7.

The Exercise
Start the exercise by taking a deep breath. As you slowly exhale, lower your neck toward your sternum and completely relax, as shown in figure 9.8.

When you are ready to inhale, gently and slowly move your chin toward the top of your left shoulder, holding the contraction until the end of your inhalation, as shown in figure 9.9.

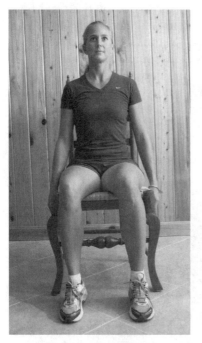
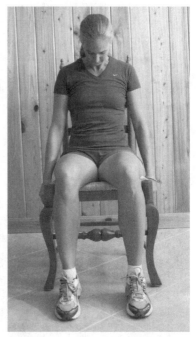

Figure 9.7 Neck Half Rolls Exercise, starting position.   *Figure 9.8 Neck Half Rolls Exercise, forward position.*

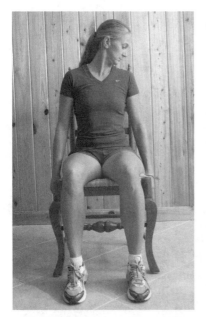

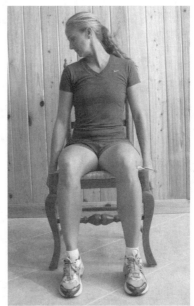

Figure 9.9 Neck Half Rolls
Exercise, left shoulder
position.

Figure 9.10 Neck Half Rolls
Exercise, right shoulder
position.

Then, as you start to exhale, lower your chin toward your breastbone, back to the forward position as shown in figure 9.8. Upon your next inhalation, move your chin toward the tip of the opposite shoulder, as shown in figure 9.10.

Repeat this exercise 3 times in the early aspect of your exercise regimen, building up to 5 repetitions by the end of your beginning exercise program.

SHOULDER EXERCISES

These exercises will strengthen your shoulder muscles, so that you can stabilize your upper torso and your arms more easily. This in turn will facilitate your riding seat regardless of your gait.

Shoulder Shrug Exercise

Starting Position
Sitting comfortably on a chair, leave your hands hanging loosely at your sides and tuck your chin slightly in, as shown in figure 9.11.

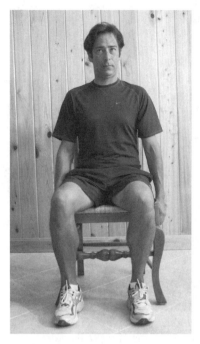 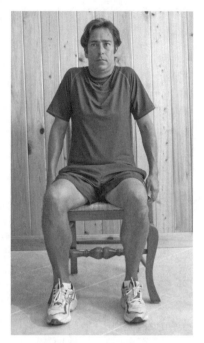

Figure 9.11 Shoulder Shrug
Exercise, starting position.

Figure 9.12 Shoulder Shrug
Exercise, ending position.

The Exercise

Start the exercise by taking a deep breath and "shrug" the points of your shoulders toward your ears. Do not bend or tense your neck. Hold this position until you complete your full inhalation breath, as shown in figure 9.12.

As you slowly exhale, lower your shoulders back to the starting position, relaxing completely as shown in figure 9.11. Repeat 5 times in the early aspect of your exercise regimen. As you get more comfortable with this exercise, build up to 10 or 20 repetitions by the end of your beginning exercise program.

Shoulder Circumduction (Circles) Exercise

The first part of the Shoulder Circumduction (Circles) Exercise will strengthen your rotator cuff group of muscles (subscapularis, supraspinatus, and infraspinatus muscles). The second part of this exercise will engage the deltoid muscles.

Starting Position

Standing upright, slightly bend your knees. Bring your navel in and hold your arms at your sides, as shown in figure 9.13.

Figure 9.13 Shoulder
Circumduction (Circles)
Exercise, starting position.

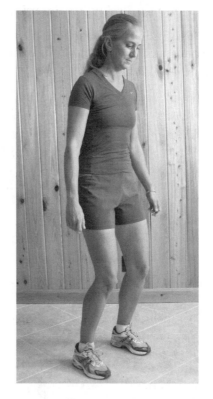

The Exercise

Start the exercise by leaning forward about 45 degrees and moving your arms in small circles, going forward 6 times followed by going backward 6 times, as shown in figure 9.14.

Next, move your arms in large circles 6 times going forward and then 6 times going backward, as shown in figure 9.15.

As you improve your practice, you can increase the number of circles performed in each direction to 20 or 25.

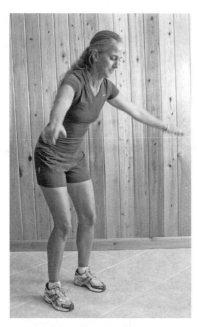

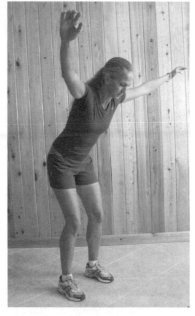

Figure 9.14 Shoulder Circumduction
(Circles) Exercise, small circles
position.

Figure 9.15 Shoulder Circumduction
(Circles) Exercise, large circles
position.

Shoulder Abduction Exercise

The Shoulder Abduction Exercise strengthens the shoulders and enhances their ability to move away from the body, as well as stabilizes the overall shoulders when needed, during sitting trot or canter for example. This in turn will help you to better stabilize your arms at all gaits and during transitions in riding.

Starting Position
While standing, take a deep breath, bring your navel in by tightening your abdominal muscles, and bend forward to engage your core muscles. Raise your arms out to your sides at shoulder level, as shown in figure 9.16.

The Exercise
Then, as you exhale, lift your arms up and back, bringing your *scapulae* (back of your shoulders) as close together as possible. Hold this position until you finish your exhalation, as shown in figure 9.17.

Finally, relax and slowly inhale while you return your arms to the starting position. Repeat 3 to 5 times in the early aspects of your exercise regimen. As you get comfortable with this exercise, build up to 10 times by the end of your beginning exercise program.

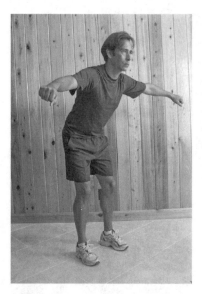

Figure 9.16 Shoulder Abduction Exercise, starting position.

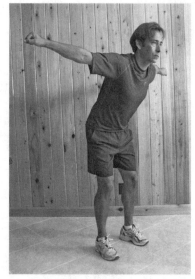

Figure 9.17 Shoulder Abduction Exercise, ending position.

Shoulder Adduction Exercise

The Shoulder Adduction Exercise helps to strengthen the shoulders and improves their ability to pull in toward the body. The exercise also contributes to a better stabilization of your arms at all gaits.

Starting Position

While standing or sitting, take a deep breath while you bring your navel in by tightening your abdominal muscles and extend your arms out in front of you with palms facing one another, as shown in figure 9.18.

The Exercise

Start the exercise by taking a deep breath. Then, as you exhale, extend your elbows out, bring your hands together, and press your palms together, as shown in figure 9.19.

Hold this position, pushing your hands against each other as hard as you can during your entire exhalation. Then relax and slowly inhale while you return your arms to the starting position. Repeat 3 to 5 times in the early aspect of your exercise regimen. Once you are comfortable with this exercise, increase your repetitions to 10 by the end of your beginning exercise program.

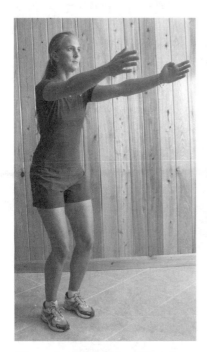 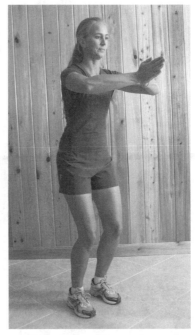

Figure 9.18 Shoulder Adduction Exercise, starting position.

Figure 9.19 Shoulder Adduction Exercise, ending position.

MID-BACK EXTENSION EXERCISE

This exercise will strengthen your entire back. A strong back is needed to maintain good posture at all gates.

If during your posture self-test you noticed that your head posture was forward and your upper back was rounded, this Mid-Back Extension Exercise will help you restore mobility and strength in your upper back, contributing to overall better posture and a better seat.

Starting Position

Lie down comfortably with your knees bent and your hands behind your neck. Place a rolled towel, 4 to 5 inches in diameter, just below your shoulder blades in the middle of your upper back as shown in figure 9.20.

The Exercise

As you start this exercise, take a deep breath and extend your back over the towel by lifting your head off the ground, but keep your hips on the floor, as shown in figure 9.21.

Your inhalation should be completed as you reach your full extension. Hold this position a few seconds. Go easy at first because it might be somewhat uncomfortable, depending on your back's stiffness.

Repeat 3 to 5 times in the early aspects of your exercise routine and increase up to 10 times by the end of your beginning exercise program.

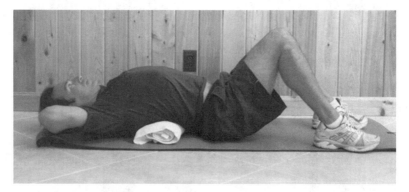

Figure 9.20 Mid-Back Extension Exercise, starting position.

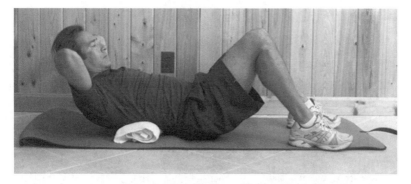

Figure 9.21 Mid-Back Extension Exercise, ending position.

STRETCHES FOR THE UPPER BODY

Stretching your upper body, neck, and shoulders right after you exercise will maintain maximum flexibility in these muscles and prevent stiffness. Because you will be warming up your body with some cardiovascular exercise prior to working out, there is no need to stretch beforehand. But you will always maximize your benefits by stretching afterward.

NECK STRETCHES

Back of the Neck Stretch

Starting Position
Lie down comfortably on your stomach with your head extending beyond the edge of a bed or a tack trunk. Hang your arms over the edge of the tack trunk, as shown in figure 9.22.

The Stretch
Start this stretch by taking a deep breath. As you slowly exhale, gently stretch your entire neck forward. Then place your hands over your head or upper neck to exert an extra push. This move will help you reach a deeper stretch, as shown in figure 9.23.

Relax in the stretch with two gentle full breaths. Feel the stretch in your back (erector spinae) muscles. Then slowly relax your stretch and bring your head back to your starting position during an exhalation.

Advanced Version of the Back of the Neck Stretch
For an advanced version of this stretch, once you get past the initial stretch, you can bring your chin towards your right or left

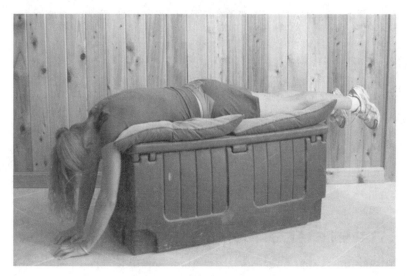

Figure 9.22 Back of the Neck Stretch, starting position.

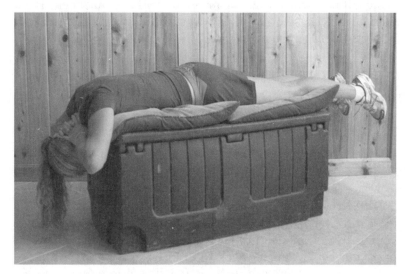

Figure 9.23 Back of the Neck Stretch, ending position.

chest. This causes an extra stretch on the opposite side of the back (erector spinae) muscle group. Take a few gentle deep breaths as you feel the stretch all along your spine.

Front of the Neck Stretch

Starting Position
Lie down comfortably on your back with your head extending beyond the edge of your bed or tack trunk. Place your arms alongside your body as shown in figure 9.24.

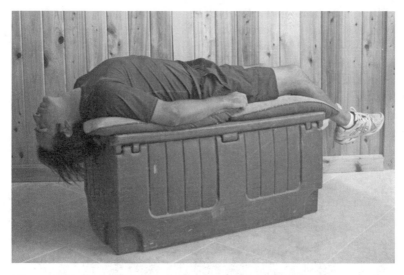

Figure 9.24 Front of the Neck Stretch, starting position.

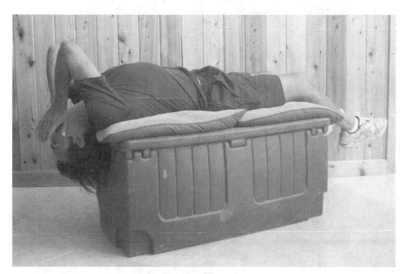

Figure 9.25 Front of the Neck Stretch, straight position.

The Stretch

Start this stretch by taking a deep breath. As you slowly exhale, relax your entire neck backward to reach the easy stretch. Then place your hands on your chin and gently push to reach progressively the deeper stretch, as shown in figure 9.25.

Then relax in the deeper stretch with a few gentle full breaths while you feel the stretch in your neck flexor muscles for at least 10 seconds. Then, during an exhalation, slowly relax your stretch and bring your head up and back to your starting position.

Advanced Version of the Front of the Neck Stretch
In the advanced version, once you get past the initial stretch you can move your chin in the direction of your right or left shoulder, as shown in figures 9.26 and 9.27. This move provides a deeper stretch on the opposite side of the neck flexor muscles. Take a few gentle deep breaths as you feel the stretch all along the sides of your neck.

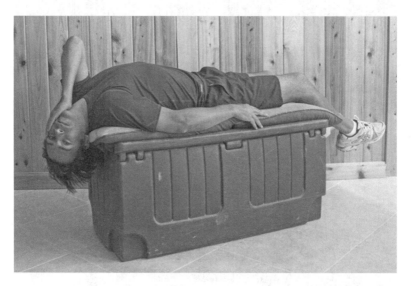

Figure 9.26 Advanced Front of the Neck Stretch, right shoulder position.

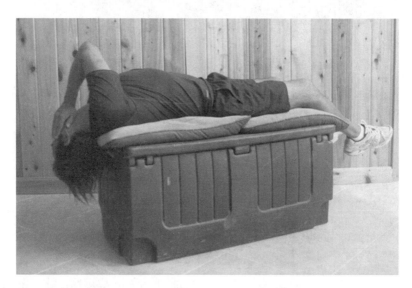

Figure 9.27 Advanced Front of the Neck Stretch, left shoulder position.

Side of the Neck Stretch

Starting Position

Lie down comfortably on your side with your head and bottom arm extending beyond the edge of your bed or tack trunk. Keep your upper arm along the side facing upward, as shown in figure 9.28.

The Stretch

Start the stretch by taking a deep breath. As you slowly exhale, relax your entire neck sideways toward the floor until you reach an easy stretch. Then, using your lower arm's hand, gently pull your head down farther toward the floor until you reach a deeper stretch, as shown in figure 9.29.

When you reach the end of the stretch, take two gentle full breaths. Feel the stretch in the muscles on the side of your neck for about 10 seconds.

Then slowly relax your stretch and bring your head up and back to your starting position during an exhalation. Roll onto your other side and repeat this stretch on the other side of your neck.

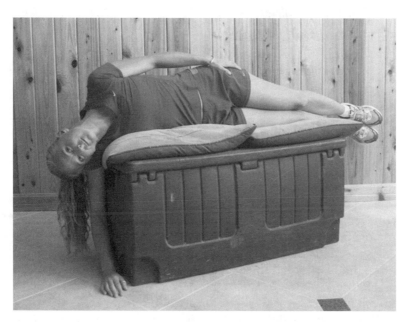

Figure 9.28 Side of the Neck Stretch, starting position.

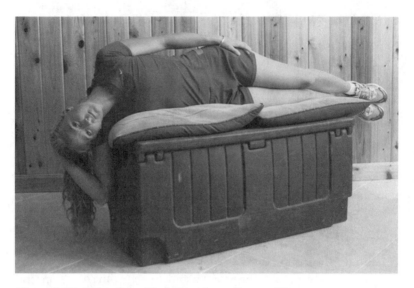

Figure 9.29 Side of the Neck Stretch, ending position.

SHOULDER STRETCHES

Back of the Shoulders Stretch

Starting Position
This Back of the Shoulders Stretch can be done sitting or stand-ing in an upright position, as shown in figure 9.30.

The Stretch
Start the stretch by taking a deep breath. Bring your right hand around to the opposite side of the neck to rest on top of your left shoulder. As you slowly exhale, bring your left hand over your bent right elbow and gently pull toward your body until you reach the easy stretch, as shown in figure 9.31.

This position will stretch your triceps, posterior deltoid, rotator cuff, teres, trapezius, and rhomboid muscles on your right side. Maintain this position for a few seconds, relaxing with two slow deep breaths. Then pull your elbow in toward your chest some more until you reach the deeper stretch. Feel the muscles loosen-ing. Please resist the temptation to jerk your arm; you could over-stretch your triceps and posterior deltoid muscles.

When you are done, slowly return to your starting position. Duplicate this stretch with your other arm.

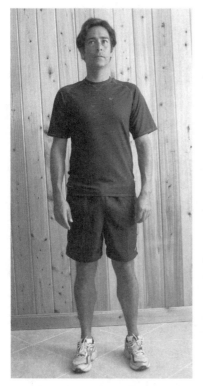
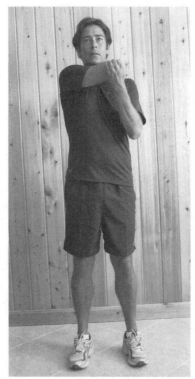

Figure 9.30 Back of the Shoulders Stretch, starting position.

Figure 9.31 Back of the Shoulders Stretch, ending position.

Front of the Shoulders Stretch

The Front of the Shoulders Stretch will stretch your biceps, pectorals, anterior deltoid, and the coracobrachialis muscles of the upper torso.

Starting Position

This stretch is best done standing. You need a door, a shelf, or simply a wall for the stretch. Start by taking a deep breath while you bring one arm behind you at shoulder height, and grab onto the door, shelf, or wall as shown in figure 9.32.

The Stretch

To start this stretch, slowly exhale and pivot your body away from the wall while slightly tightening your back arm muscle. Keep twisting until you reach an easy stretch, as shown in figure 9.33.

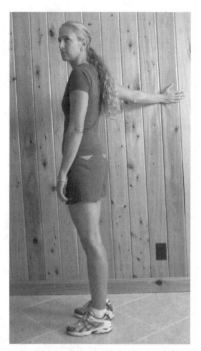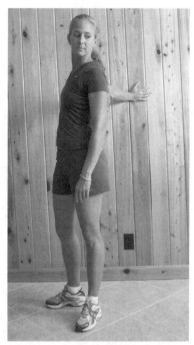

Figure 9.32 Front of the Shoulders   *Figure 9.33 Front of the Shoulders*
Stretch, starting position.   *Stretch, ending position.*

Relax in this position with a few slow breaths. Then pivot some more to reach a deeper stretch. Feel your shoulder muscles relax.

When you are done, slowly return to your starting position and duplicate this stretch with your other arm.

Simultaneous Back of the Shoulders Stretch

This stretch will extend your latissimus dorsi, deltoid, teres, rotator cuff, and rhomboid muscles of the back of your shoulders.

Starting Position
This stretch is best done while standing. You need a chair, a table, or simply a wall for this stretch. Take a deep breath while you bring both your hands to rest on the chair, table, or wall in front of you, as shown in figure 9.34.

The Stretch
To begin, slowly exhale, pull your navel in, and lean your body forward (at a 90-degree angle to the chair, table, or wall) until you reach an easy stretch, as shown in figure 9.35.

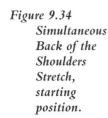

Figure 9.34
   Simultaneous
   Back of the
   Shoulders
   Stretch,
   starting
   position.

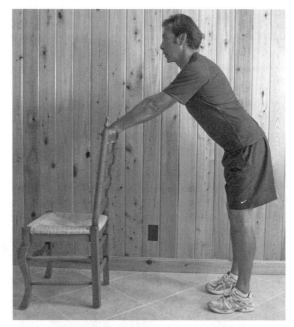

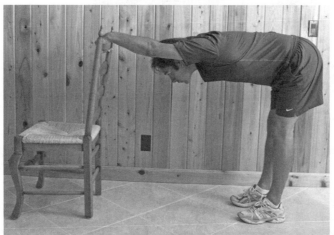

Figure 9.35 Simultaneous Back of the Shoulders Stretch, ending position.

Maintain this position while relaxing with a few slow breaths. Then lean farther to reach a deeper stretch. Feel the muscles begin to relax.

When you are done, slowly return to your starting position.

Simultaneous Front of the Shoulders Stretch

This stretch will extend your pectoral, biceps, anterior deltoid, and rotator cuff muscles of the front of your shoulders.

Starting Position

This is a standing stretch. You need a doorframe for this stretch. Extend your arms and hold onto the doorframe, as shown in figure 9.36.

The Stretch

Start the stretch by taking a deep breath. Then as you slowly exhale, pull your navel in, take a step forward, and lean your upper body forward until you reach an easy stretch, as shown in figure 9.37.

Maintain this position for about 20 seconds while relaxing with a few slow full breaths. Then lean forward some more until you reach the deeper stretch. Feel your muscles letting go.

When you are done, return to your starting position.

Advanced Version of the Front of the Shoulders Stretch

For an advanced version of the Front of the Shoulders Stretch, you can raise or lower your hand position as you please. This will change the actual location of the stretch over your anterior chest and arm muscles, giving you a chance to focus your efforts where you need it the most.

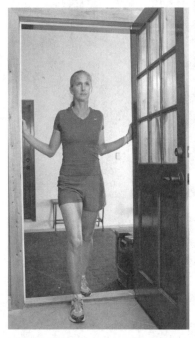 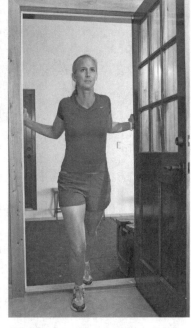

Figure 9.36 Simultaneous Front of the Shoulders Stretch, starting position.

Figure 9.37 Simultaneous Front of the Shoulders Stretch, ending position.

10

LOWER BODY EXERCISES AND STRETCHES

Possessing a strong lower body is important because it directly assists you with your balance when riding. Your legs wrap themselves around the horse's chest, providing stability during transitional gaits. In order to stay on top of the horse's center of gravity, the lower body must constantly provide stability to the core muscles. Tension in your lower body leads to buttock and leg stiffness, possible cramps, and eventually pain. A strong lower body contributes to good posture, stability, athletic performance, and finesse of execution when riding.

By lower body, I mean the hips and legs. (See figures 2.3 through 2.5 in chapter 2 for illustrations of these muscles.) The following are considered lower-body muscles:

Hip Muscles

- The gluteal muscles (hip retractor muscles)
- The iliopsoas muscles (hip flexor muscles)

Leg Muscles

- The adductor muscles
- The calf muscles and hamstring muscles (leg retractor muscles)
- The quadriceps muscles and shin muscles (leg extensor muscles)

The hips perform flexion and extension movements. The legs perform flexion, extension, adduction, abduction, and circumduction movements.

Some great exercises that will quickly and safely develop your lower body musculature are listed in this chapter. Stretches that will help you maintain maximum flexibility in these muscles are also discussed. Because you will warm up with some cardiovascular exercises presented in chapter 7, there is no need to stretch before your workout. However, you should stretch afterward to loosen your muscles and prevent stiffness.

STRENGTHENING EXERCISES FOR THE LOWER BODY

HIP EXERCISES

For a good seat, strong hip flexor (iliopsoas) muscles are essential. Hip flexor muscles govern the action between the thighs and the hips. This, combined with the good use of your core muscles and other leg muscles, will help you secure a good seat during any motion.

Hip Flexion Exercise

The Hip Flexion Exercise will activate the hip flexor muscles (iliopsoas) as well as the lower abdominals.

Starting Position
Lying comfortably on your back, place your hands under your head. Flex your knees and cross your legs by placing one of your ankles over the other one, as shown in figure 10.1.

The Exercise
Start the exercise by taking a deep breath. As you slowly exhale, lift your knees up toward your head. Through your entire breath maintain the contraction and try to bring your knees as close to your head as you can, lifting your pelvis away from the floor, as shown in figure 10.2.

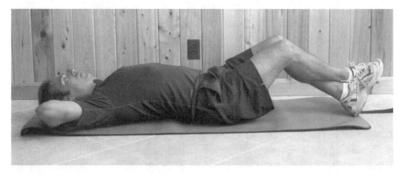

Figure 10.1 Hip Flexion Exercise, starting position.

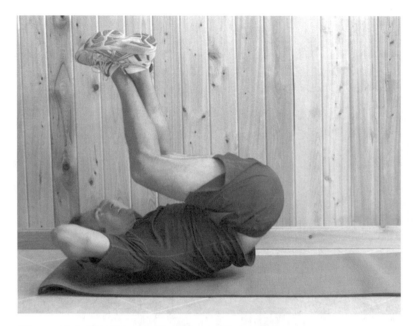

Figure 10.2 Hip Flexion Exercise, ending position.

As you reach your full contraction, hold for 2 seconds. Then relax by slowly inhaling while lowering your hips until your lower back and feet touch the floor. Repeat this exercise 3 to 5 times in the early aspects of your exercise routine. By the end of your beginning exercise program, you should be strong enough to easily perform 10 repetitions in one session.

Hip Extension Exercise

The Hip Extension Exercise will activate the back (erector spinae), the sacrospinalis (lower back), and the gluteal muscles.

Starting Position
Lying comfortably on your stomach, place the palms of your hands on the floor alongside your lower rib cage, as shown in figure 10.3.

The Exercise
Start the exercise by taking a deep breath. As you slowly exhale, lift your head, chest, and legs off the ground. Your knees should lift off the floor. Maintain the contraction through your entire breath, using your arms to assist you at the end of the range, as shown in figure 10.4.

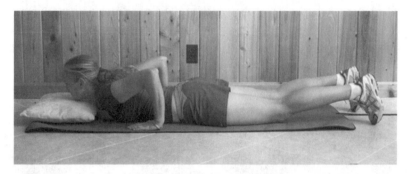

Figure 10.3 Hip Extension Exercise, starting position.

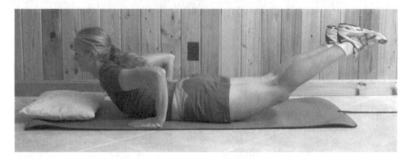

Figure 10.4 Hip Extension Exercise, ending position.

As you reach your full contraction, hold for 2 seconds. Then relax by slowly inhaling while lowering your chest and legs until you are lying down on the floor again. Repeat this exercise 3 to 5 times in the early aspects of your exercise regimen. You should be able to easily handle 10 repetitions of this exercise by the end of your beginning exercise program.

LEG EXERCISES

Leg Flexion and Extension: The Leg Squat Exercise

The Leg Squat Exercise will strengthen both the quadriceps and hamstrings.

Starting Position
Stand with your feet shoulder-width apart, bring your navel in, and raise your arms to shoulder level, as shown in figure 10.5.

The Exercise
Start the exercise by taking a deep breath as you gently bend your knees and lower your body until your gluteals almost touch your ankles, as shown in figure 10.6.

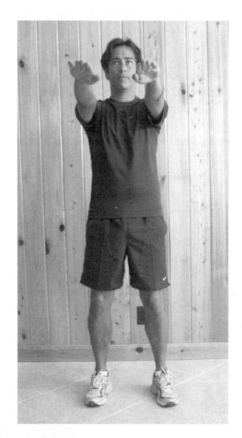

Figure 10.5 Leg Squat Exercise, starting position.

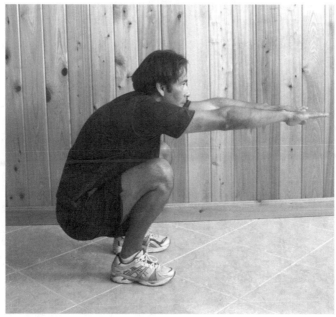

Figure 10.6 Leg Squat Exercise, ending position.

Then as you exhale, rise back up to the starting position. Repeat 5 times at the start of your exercise routine. By the end of the beginning exercise program, you should be able to easily perform 10 repetitions.

Advanced Version of the Leg Squat Exercise

The Advanced Leg Squat Exercise will increase the workload of your legs. First assume the starting position of the Leg Squat Exercise, but put a thick telephone book underneath your heels, as shown in figure 10.7.

The phone book changes the angle of your ankles and increases the mechanical stress on both the flexor and extensor muscle groups of your legs while performing the squat, as shown in figure 10.8.

To increase the strengthening benefit of this exercise, twist your torso to either the right or the left as you push upward, as shown respectively in figures 10.9 and 10.10.

When doing the Advanced Leg Squat Exercise, consider starting the exercise by going straight up and down for a few repetitions until you feel a light "burn" in your legs, then alternate twisting to the right or to the left as you please. This movement accentuates the benefit of this workout to both your core and leg muscles.

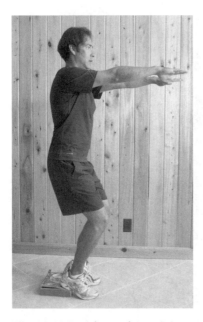 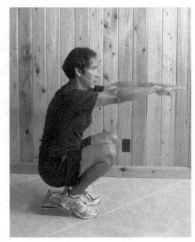

Figure 10.7 Advanced Leg Squat
Exercise, starting position.

Figure 10.8 Advanced Leg Squat
Exercise, squatting.

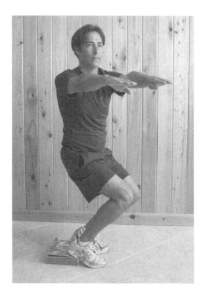

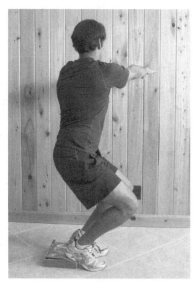

Figure 10.9 Advanced Leg Squat Exercise, right position.

Figure 10.10 Advanced Leg Squat Exercise, left position.

Leg Abduction Exercise

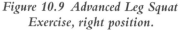

The Leg Abduction Exercise will activate the gluteal muscles as well as the lower abdominals. Strengthening the muscles responsible for leg abduction will contribute to a better control over your seat at all gaits and during transitional movements.

Starting Position

The Leg Abduction Exercise is best done while standing. However, you need a chair, table, or simply a wall to help you stay balanced, as shown in figure 10.11.

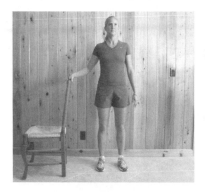

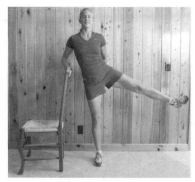

Figure 10.11 Leg Abduction Exercise, starting position.

Figure 10.12 Leg Abduction Exercise, ending position.

The Exercise

Start the exercise by taking a deep breath while you grasp the chair with your right hand to stay balanced. Bring your navel in. Then, as you slowly exhale, lift your left leg to the side as high as you can, as shown in figure 10.12. Hold your leg in this position until you finish your exhalation.

You should be able to bring your leg almost parallel to the floor, 90 degrees from your right leg. Repeat this exercise 3 to 5 times in the early part of your exercise regimen. As you get stronger, you should be able to build up to 10 repetitions by the time you reach the end of your beginning exercise program.

Leg Adduction Exercise

The Leg Adduction Exercise will activate the adductor muscles of your legs. Strengthening these muscles will contribute to a stronger leg contact with your horse's chest, resulting in a better control of your seat when riding.

Starting Position

To begin the Leg Adduction Exercise, lie down comfortably on your back with your knees flexed and arms by your sides. Place a pillow underneath your neck and a rolled towel between your knees, as shown in figure 10.13.

The Exercise

Start the exercise by taking a deep breath and pulling your navel in. Then squeeze your knees together as you slowly exhale. Hold the contraction through the entire breath, as shown in figure 10.14.

When you are done, relax as you inhale. Repeat this exercise 3 to 5 times in the early part of your exercise routine. By the end of your beginning exercise program, you should be able to do 10 repetitions of this leg exercise.

STRETCHES FOR THE LOWER BODY

The following stretches will help you keep your lower body flexible at all times. When you build muscle, stiffness is often a side effect that affects the range of motion of the various joints of the lower body. These stretches will erase that stiffness and maximize your flexibility, which will in turn assist in the finesse of executing a good seat.

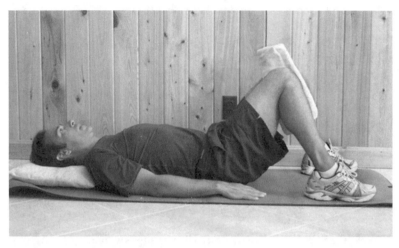

Figure 10.13 Leg Adduction Exercise, starting position.

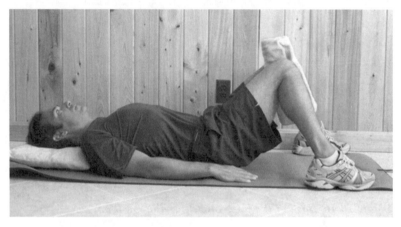

Figure 10.14 Leg Adduction Exercise, ending position.

HIP STRETCHES

Back of the Hips Stretch

The Back of the Hips Stretch affects the back (erector spinae) and gluteal muscles.

Starting Position

Lying comfortably on your back, bend your knees and keep them shoulder-width apart. Then place the palms of your hands on the back of your thighs above the knees, as shown in figure 10.15.

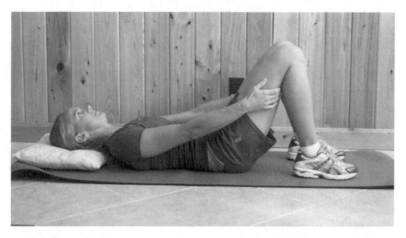

Figure 10.15 Back of the Hips Stretch, starting position.

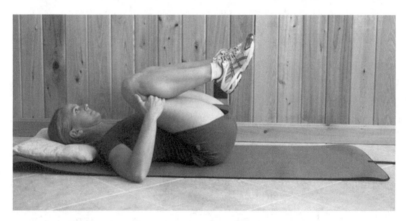

Figure 10.16 Back of the Hips Stretch, ending position.

The Stretch

To begin the stretch, take a deep breath. As you slowly exhale, lift your knees toward your armpits until you feel the easy stretch over the lower back muscles. Hold this stretch for 10 to 15 seconds to give your muscles, ligaments, and fascia time to relax as shown in figure 10.16.

Relax with a few full breaths. Then lift your knees some more to reach the deeper stretch. Feel your back muscles letting go. When done, relax by slowly inhaling while lowering your knees until your lower back and feet touch the floor.

Front of the Hips Stretch

The Front of the Hips Stretch will affect the abdominal and hip flexor muscles.

Starting Position
Lying comfortably on your stomach, place the palms of your hands on the floor by your armpits, as shown in figure 10.17. You may want to place a small pillow under your chin.

The Stretch
To begin the stretch, take a deep breath. As you slowly exhale, gently push up your upper body with your arms until you reach the easy stretch and you feel the bones of your hips lift from the floor. Once at that point, hold the stretch for 10 to 15 seconds to give your muscles, ligaments, and fascia time to relax as shown in figure 10.18.

Relax with a few full breaths. Then consider arching your back some more to reach the deeper stretch; however, keep your

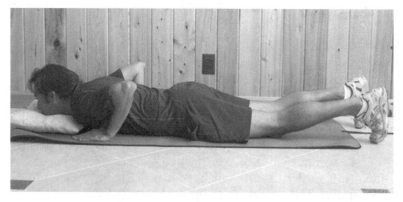

Figure 10.17 Front of the Hips Stretch, starting position.

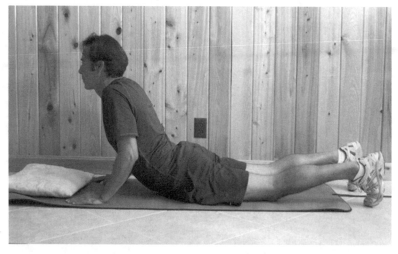

Figure 10.18 Front of the Hips Stretch, ending position.

hipbones touching the floor. When you are done, relax by slowly inhaling and lower your body back to the floor.

LEG STRETCHES

Back of the Legs Stretch

The Back of the Legs Stretch targets the hamstrings and calf muscles of your legs.

Starting Position

This stretch is done while lying on your back. You will need a long towel. Bend the leg you are about to stretch and hold the towel around your foot like it's in a sling. If your back is tight, you might consider flexing your other knee slightly to relieve the pressure on your back. Hold the two ends of the towel with your hands, as shown in figure 10.19.

The Stretch

Start the stretch by taking a deep breath. As you gently exhale, slowly straighten your leg until you feel the easy stretch over your calf and hamstrings, as shown in figure 10.20.

For a deeper stretch, when you reach the full knee extension gradually move your knee towards your chest by contracting your quadriceps and pulling on your towel. Maintain this position for 10 to 15 seconds while relaxing with a few slow deep breaths, as shown in figure 10.21. If your back is really tight, your buttocks may lift off the floor and your opposite leg may bend at the knee. These movements are simply compensating in proportion to the tension in the back.

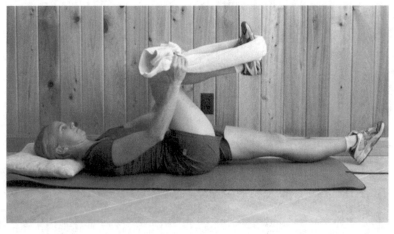

Figure 10.19 Back of the Legs Stretch, starting position.

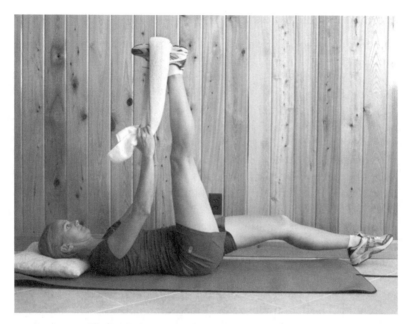

Figure 10.20 Back of the Legs Stretch, ending position.

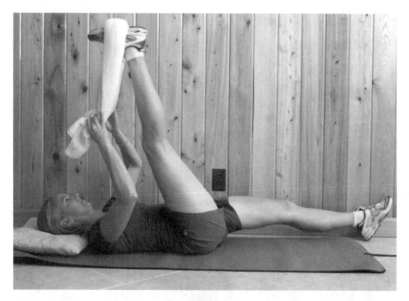

Figure 10.21 Back of the Legs Stretch, the deeper stretch.

When you are done, flex your knee and return to your starting position. Duplicate this stretch with your opposite leg.

Front of the Legs Stretch

The Front of the Legs Stretch will target your quadriceps and shin muscles.

Starting Position

This stretch is best done while lying on your side, with the side to be stretched facing up, as shown in figure 10.22.

The Stretch

Start the stretch by taking a deep breath while pulling in your navel. Move your uppermost leg behind you and gently grab your ankle with your hand. If you can't reach your ankle, use a towel as a sling around your ankle. Gently move your ankle backward as you contract your hamstrings and gluteals until you reach the easy stretch, as shown in figure 10.23.

Maintain this position for 10 to 15 seconds, relaxing with a few slow deep breaths. Then pull some more to reach the deeper stretch. Feel your muscles relax.

When you are done, slowly return to your starting position. Roll over to your other side and duplicate this stretch with the other leg.

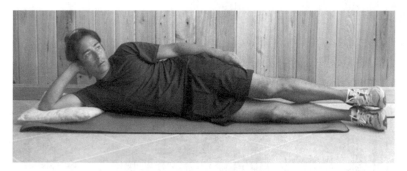

Figure 10.22 Front of the Legs Stretch, starting position.

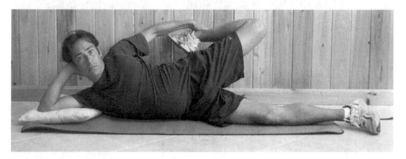

Figure 10.23 Front of the Legs Stretch, ending position.

Adductors of the Legs Stretch

The Adductors of the Legs Stretch will target your adductor muscle group, which is responsible for pulling the leg toward the body.

Starting Position

This stretch is best done while standing and using a chair or a bed. Lift the leg to be stretched, extend it, and place it comfortably on the chair to create the easy stretch, as shown in figure 10.24.

The Stretch

To begin the stretch, take a deep breath and pull your navel in. Then as you exhale slowly, gently flex your *other* (standing) leg to create a deeper stretch of your adductor muscles, as shown in figure 10.25. Adjust your position until you reach a comfortable stretching position.

Maintain this position, relaxing with a few slow breaths. When you are done, slowly return to your starting position. Duplicate this stretch with your other leg.

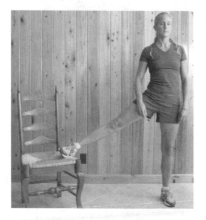 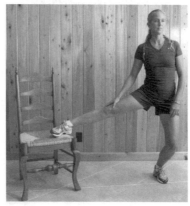

Figure 10.24 Adductors of the Legs Stretch, starting position.   *Figure 10.25 Adductors of the Legs Stretch, ending position.*

Abductors of the Legs Stretch

The Abductors of the Legs Stretch will target your abductor muscles, which are responsible for moving the leg away from the body.

Starting Position

This stretch is done while standing beside a wall or a chair so you can maintain your balance. Cross the leg to be stretched in front and past the midline of your body to reach the easy stretch, as shown in figure 10.26.

The Stretch

To begin, take a deep breath and pull your navel in. As you exhale slowly, gently lower your body toward the floor to reach the deeper stretch, as shown in figure 10.27. Adjust your stretch until you reach a comfortable position.

Maintain this position, relaxing with a few slow breaths. When done, slowly return to your starting position. Duplicate this stretch with your other leg.

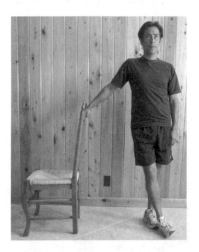   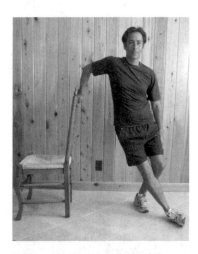

Figure 10.26 Abductors of the Legs Stretch, starting position.   *Figure 10.27 Abductors of the Legs Stretch, ending position.*

11

This chapter presents some very simple exercises to help you strengthen your overall coordination between the core, upper, and lower muscle groups.

GENERAL EXTENSION EXERCISE

The General Extension Exercise will strengthen the back muscles that help you maintain proper posture in your seat.

STARTING POSITION

Lie comfortably on your stomach, with your arms relaxed and extended above your head. Keep your chin tucked in so that your neck stays in a neutral position, as shown in figure 11.1. You may want to place a small pillow under your chin and chest.

THE EXERCISE

To begin the exercise, take a deep breath through your nose. As you start exhaling, simultaneously lift your upper body, arms, and legs off the floor a few inches. Rotate your arms so that your hands point up to the ceiling. Squeeze your gluteals as you lift your legs. Keep them squeezed throughout the entire exercise, as shown in figure 11.2.

Make sure you don't overextend your neck. Keep it in line with your torso by keeping your chin slightly tucked in. In your early practice of this exercise, start easy by only lifting your body a couple inches and holding that position for about 10 seconds or three deep breaths. As you progress with this exercise, try to lift a little higher, up to 5 inches, and hold a little longer, up to 20 seconds.

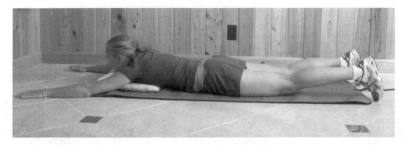

Figure 11.1 General Extension Exercise, starting position.

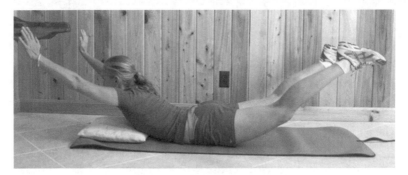

Figure 11.2 General Extension Exercise, ending position.

GENERAL FLEXION EXERCISE

The General Flexion Exercise will strengthen the anterior muscles of the neck, arms, abdomen, hips, and legs, which will help you hold your seat with greater ease.

STARTING POSITION

Lie comfortably on your back, arms relaxed along your sides. Tuck your chin in, as shown in figure 11.4.

THE EXERCISE

Begin the exercise by taking a deep breath through your nose. As you start exhaling, simultaneously lift your upper body, arms, and legs off the floor a few inches. For maximum benefits, point your fingers and toes straight ahead, and keep your chin slightly tucked, as shown in figure 11.4.

In your early practice of this exercise, start easy by only lifting your body and legs a couple of inches and holding that position for about 10 seconds. As you progress with your exercise program, try to lift your feet and arms higher and hold longer, up to a maximum of 30 seconds.

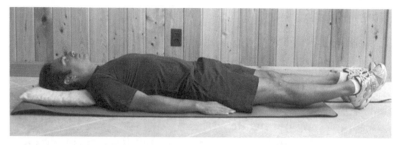

Figure 11.3 General Flexion Exercise, starting position.

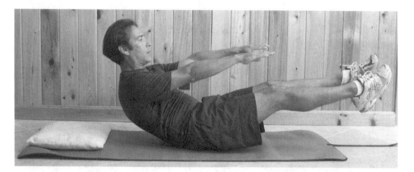

Figure 11.4 General Flexion Exercise, ending position.

THE TWIST EXERCISE

The Twist Exercise is a cardiovascular exercise that engages your abdominal wall muscles. Performing this exercise several times will help to loosen your hips, lower back, and abdominal muscles.

STARTING POSITION

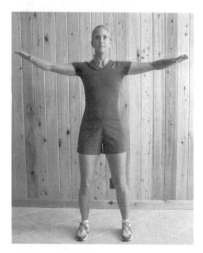

Stand relaxed with your feet shoulder-width apart and raise your arms out to the side to shoulder height, as shown in figure 11.5. You can extend or flex your forearms if you like, but keep your elbows at shoulder height during the entire exercise.

Figure 11.5 The Twist Exercise, starting position.

THE EXERCISE

To start this exercise, you will twist to loosen your waistline. Rotate your upper body to the left so you face 90 degrees from your starting position, as shown in figure 11.6.

Next, return to your starting position and then turn your upper body to the right so you are facing 90 degrees from the starting position, as shown in figure 11.7.

You can repeat the entire Twist Exercise slowly a couple more times to really loosen your muscles. Then slightly increase the rhythm and repeat 10 times.

ADVANCED TWIST EXERCISE

Next, increase your workout by performing the Advanced Twist Exercise. You begin in the same starting position as the Twist Exercise, but you will lift each knee to the opposite side. So when you rotate to the left, lift the left knee up and toward the right elbow, as shown in figure 11.8.

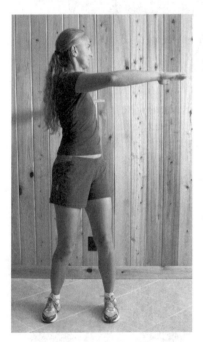 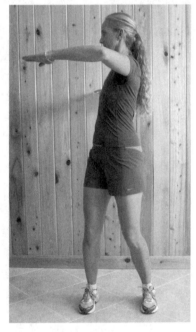

Figure 11.6 The Twist Exercise, left position.   *Figure 11.7 The Twist Exercise, right position.*

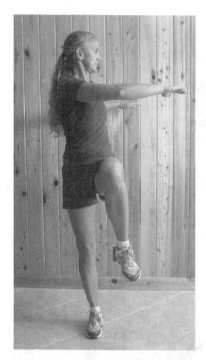 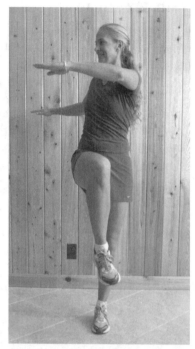

*Figure 11.8 Advanced Twist
Exercise, left knee to the
right elbow position.*

*Figure 11.9 Advanced Twist
Exercise, right knee to the
left elbow position.*

Then, when rotating to the right, lift your right knee up and toward the left elbow, as shown in figure 11.9.

Repeat 20 to 30 times on each side to really exercise your core muscles.

THE BRIDGE EXERCISE

The Bridge Exercise requires the combined effort of many of your core muscles.

STARTING POSITION

Lie comfortably on your back and relax your spine, but don't overarch or push your lower back against the floor. You may place a small pillow underneath your neck. Keep your arms at your sides and bend your knees, as shown in figure 11.10.

THE EXERCISE

Start this exercise by taking a deep breath through your nose. Then bring your navel in while contracting your transversus abdominis muscle by coughing. As you hold the contraction, start exhaling and raise your hips off the floor. Sustain your abdominal contraction until you reach the position where your hips are in line with your thighs and shoulders, as shown in figure 11.11.

Hold this position for about 8 seconds or two deep breaths. When done, relax and return to your starting position. You can repeat this entire Bridge Exercise 5 times in your beginning exercise program. Build up to 10 repetitions over the course of a month.

Consider increasing your workout by lifting and extending one of your legs while holding the bridge position, as shown in figure 11.12. Then perform the exercise again, but lift the opposite leg.

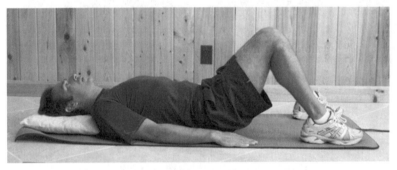

Figure 11.10 The Bridge Exercise, starting position.

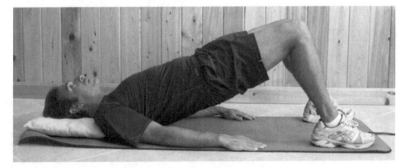

Figure 11.11 The Bridge Exercise, hips aligned with shoulders and thighs.

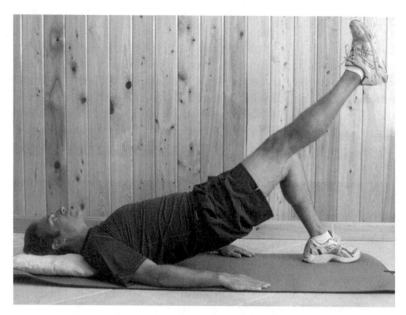

Figure 11.12 The Bridge Exercise, hips aligned and extending one leg.

KNEE SQUEEZE EXERCISE

The Knee Squeeze Exercise requires the combined effort of many of your core muscles.

STARTING POSITION

Lie on your back with your spine relaxed, without overarching or pushing your lower back against the floor. Keep your arms at your sides and bend your knees. Place a small rolled towel between your knees and firmly squeeze them together, as shown in figure 11.13.

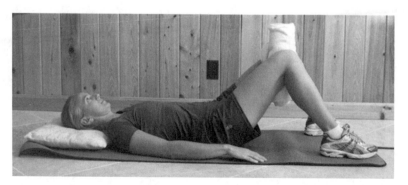

Figure 11.13 The Knee Squeeze Exercise, starting position.

THE EXERCISE

Start the exercise by taking a deep breath through your nose. Then pull your navel in and contract your transversus abdominis muscles by coughing. As you hold the contraction in your abdominal muscles, start exhaling and lower both knees to the right side, as shown in figure 11.14. Keep squeezing your knees throughout the entire movement. Go as far as you can without any discomfort. You should feel a stretch in your left abdominal muscles. Relax and inhale.

Using the core muscles on your left side, gently pull your knees back up as you exhale. Keep squeezing your knees throughout the entire movement. When you return to your starting position, repeat the same exercise on the left side. You can repeat the entire Knee Squeeze Exercise (both sides) 5 times in your beginning exercise program. Build up to 10 repetitions over the course of a month.

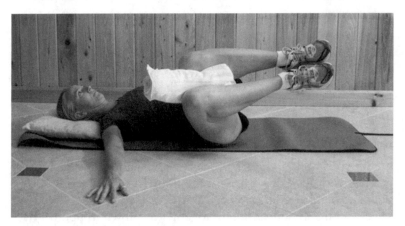

Figure 11.14 The Knee Squeeze Exercise, right position.

12

The beginner exercise program is designed to progressively help you get started on developing a better seat. This workout schedule gently gets your muscle groups going without the risk of hurting yourself. Within ten days you will feel a great improvement in your body awareness of your seat and a much better control of your overall posture.

As you progress in this program, you will become fitter and these exercises will become easier to perform. From this simple beginner program you will feel a great improvement in the use of your core muscles, which will directly result in a better seat.

This beginning exercise program starts with breathing exercises, followed by a short overall body warm-up. Then your exercise routine progresses by working your core muscles and upper body, and finishes with a lower-body workout.

BREATHING EXERCISES

Developing a full breath right from the start of this program is critical. Practice the **Full Breath Exercise** from chapter 3 (see figures 3.1 through 3.3) at least once a day (12 repetitions) for the first ten days of your beginning program. Do not hesitate to practice this particular exercise at any time in your day-to-day life to stretch your entire breathing apparatus and release deep tensions in your inner fascia and muscle layers. As you know, practice makes perfect, and it is to your advantage if taking a full breath becomes second nature. This way, every time you feel stressed or panicky, your reflex will be to take several full breaths to calm down and to get more oxygen to your brain. A great benefit to taking full breaths is that it helps you stay alert and connected to reality. Remember, if you use your full breath, you use your full brain.

Next, you will focus on developing a strong diaphragm muscle. Practice the **Diaphragm Breathing Exercise** from chapter 3 (see figures 3.4 through 3.6) at least once a day (10 repetitions) for the first ten days of your exercise program. You will be amazed by the benefits of this practice. Whenever you feel tired or sluggish, this exercise is the quickest way to feel revitalized due to the increased oxygen levels in your lungs. I personally practice this exercise every day with 5 to 10 repetitions, and sometimes I perform it several times a day. With practice you will begin to realize how this breathing exercise also helps relax the core muscles.

WARM UP YOUR BODY

Use the exercises in chapter 7 to warm up your body before you begin specific body exercises. Start with the easy version of the **Walking on the Spot Exercise** (see figures 7.1 through 7.5), where you simply bring your knee up to 90 degrees from your trunk. Your pace should be to lift a knee every 3 seconds. Two to three minutes of this exercise is sufficient to get your body warmed up. Then follow with the easy version of the **Arm Twist Exercise** (see figures 7.11 through 7.13) where you simply rotate your upper body to each side. Repeat each side 5 times.

After three days, consider moving to the **Advanced Arm Twist Exercise** (see figures 7.14 and 7.15) where you bring your knees up as you rotate your upper body to the opposite side. Repeat the exercise 5 times on each side.

CORE MUSCLES WORKOUT

Now you will begin to exercise by performing the core muscle exercises from chapter 8. Start practicing the easy version of the **Abdominal Muscles Exercise** (see figures 8.1 through 8.3) for 6 repetitions. Take your time when performing this exercise to really feel your abdominal muscles working.

Then move on to the **Back Muscles Exercise** (see figures 8.6 and 8.7) for 6 repetitions. Again, take your time during this exercise to feel your back muscles working.

Next you need to stretch your core muscles. So, while you are lying on your stomach from the preceding exercise, move on to the **Abdominal Muscles Stretch** (see figures 8.8 and 8.9). Do not rush. Feel the stretch deep in your abdominal wall.

Finally, move on to stretch your back with the **Back Muscles Stretch** (see figures 8.10 and 8.11). Again, take your time so you can feel the stretch deep along your spine.

UPPER BODY WORKOUT

The next phase of your beginner exercise program targets the upper body with exercises from chapter 9. Start working your upper body by practicing the **Neck Half Rolls Exercise** (see figures 9.7 through 9.10) for 5 to 10 repetitions. Take your time during this exercise so you can feel your neck muscles working.

Follow with the **Shoulder Shrug Exercise** (see figures 9.11 and 9.12). Start this exercise slowly to really feel the trapezius muscles working. Increase your rhythm as you proceed. By the end of the ten days, you should be able to complete 20 repetitions.

Then proceed with the **Shoulder Circumduction (Circles) Exercise** (see figures 9.13 through 9.15). Move slowly so you can feel every muscle being stretched as you perform this exercise. Perform 6 circles.

When finished with these exercises, practice these neck stretches in the following order:

1. The **Back of the Neck Stretch** (see figures 9.22 and 9.23), gently and progressively stretching the back extensor muscles.
2. The **Front of the Neck Stretch** (see figures 9.24 through 9.27), gently and progressively stretching the neck flexors. Include the advanced version of this stretch.
3. The **Side of the Neck Stretch** (see figures 9.28 and 9.29), gently and progressively stretching the side neck muscles.

Follow with the shoulder stretches, in this order:

1. The **Simultaneous Back of the Shoulders Stretch** (see figure 9.34 and 9.35), gently and progressively stretching the back of the shoulders.
2. The **Simultaneous Front of the Shoulders Stretch** (see figures 9.36 and 9.37), gently and progressively stretching the chest and upper-arm muscles.

LOWER BODY WORKOUT

The final phase of the beginning exercise program utilizes lower-body exercises from chapter 10. Start with the **Hip Flexion Exercise** (see figures 10.1 and 10.2) for 3 to 5 repetitions. Take your time during this exercise to feel your hip flexor muscles working.

Follow with the **Hip Extension Exercise** (see figures 10.3 and 10.4). Allow yourself to feel your hip extensor muscles really working. Repeat this exercise 3 times until you are able to lift your knees easily off the floor.

Finish your routine with the **Leg Squat Exercise** (see figures 10.5 and 10.6). Take your time during this exercise so you can feel both your leg flexor and extensor muscles working. Make sure you go all the way down, so your buttocks touch your heels. Repeat 5 times.

When done with these exercises, move on to stretching your lower body, starting with these hip stretches:

1. The **Back of the Hips Stretch** (see figures 10.15 and 10.16), gently and progressively stretching the back of the hips.
2. The **Front of the Hips Stretch** (see figures 10.17 and 10.18), gently and progressively stretching the front of the hips.

End with these leg stretches, in the following order:

1. The **Back of the Legs Stretch** (see figures 10.19 through 10.21), gently and progressively stretching the back of the legs.
2. The **Front of the Legs Stretch** (see figures 10.22 and 10.23), gently and progressively stretching the front of the legs.

BEGINNING EXERCISE PROGRAM CHART

You can use the following chart as a reference when performing the beginning exercise program outlined in this chapter. The exercises are presented in sequential order beginning with the breathing exercises and ending with the final stretch of the lower body. You should be able to perform the suggested number of repetitions by the end of the 10 days. You can use this chart as a quick reference once you start incorporating this beginning exercise program into your daily routine. Good luck with your new workout!

BEGINNING EXERCISE PROGRAM CHART
(15-MINUTE ROUTINE)

ORDER OF EXERCISES	EXERCISE OR STRETCH	REPETITIONS	TIME
1	Full Breath Exercise	12	3 minutes
2	Diaphragm Breathing Exercise	10	20 seconds
3	Walking on the Spot Exercise	30	2–3 minutes
4	Arm Twist Exercise	5	15 seconds
5	Advanced Arm Twist Exercise	5	15 seconds
6	Abdominal Muscles Exercise	6	1 minute
7	Back Muscles Exercise	6	1 minute
8	Abdominal Muscles Stretch	1	30 seconds
9	Back Muscles Stretch	1	30 seconds
10	Neck Half Rolls Exercise	5–10	50 seconds
11	Shoulder Shrug Exercise	20	15 seconds
12	Shoulder Circumduction (Circles) Exercise	6	15 seconds
13	Back of the Neck Stretch	1	20 seconds
14	Front of the Neck Stretch	1	20 seconds
15	Side of the Neck Stretch x 2	1	30 seconds
16	Simultaneous Back of the Shoulders Stretch	1	30 seconds

(continued)

	BEGINNING EXERCISE PROGRAM CHART (CONTINUED)		
ORDER OF EXERCISES	EXERCISE OR STRETCH	REPETITIONS	TIME
17	Simultaneous Front of the Shoulders Stretch	1	20 seconds
18	Hip Flexion Exercise	3–5	40 seconds
19	Hip Extension Exercise	3	40 seconds
20	Leg Squat Exercise	5	1 minute
21	Back of the Hips Stretch	1	30 seconds
22	Front of the Hips Stretch	1	30 seconds
23	Back of the Legs Stretch	1	30 seconds
24	Front of the Legs Stretch	1	30 seconds

13

The intermediate exercise program is designed to help you strengthen your body over the next twenty days of your exercise regimen. This workout schedule will help you develop strong core muscles as well as the muscles of your upper and lower body. Regular practice will make this program feel easier every day. Soon you will experience a stronger control of your core, upper body, and lower body muscles, leading to an overall better seat.

The intermediate exercise program begins with warm-up exercises, followed by workouts of the upper and lower body. A chart covering all of the exercises employed in this intermediate workout concludes the chapter. All of the intermediate exercises and stretches are also shown as thumbnail figures on the accompanying foldout sheets, which you can tear out and use as a handy reference.

Warm Up Your Body

Start the intermediate exercise program by performing several warm-up exercises from chapter 7. Begin with the **Advanced Walking on the Spot Exercise** (see figures 7.6 and 7.7) where you bring your knee up to the opposite side of your chest. Your pace should be to lift a knee every 3 seconds, but closer to 2 seconds if you can manage it. Two minutes of this exercise will be more than sufficient to get your body warmed up.

Follow with the **Scissor Feet Exercise** (see figures 7.8 through 7.10) for 25 repetitions.

Then move on to perform several core-muscle exercises from chapter 8.

Continue your routine with the **Abdominal Muscles Exercise** (see figures 8.1 through 8.3) for 6 repetitions and then switch to the **Advanced Abdominal Muscles Exercise** for another 6 repetitions (see figures 8.4 and 8.5).

Finish your exercise routine with the **Back Muscles Exercise** (see figures 8.6 and 8.7) for 10 repetitions. Take your time when doing this exercise so that you can feel your back muscles working. The curve your back makes when performing this exercise should become more obvious as you progress with your workout.

When done, relax for a few breaths. Then, move on to stretch your upper body, beginning with the **Abdominal Muscles Stretch** (see figures 8.8 and 8.9). Do not rush; feel the stretch deep in your abdominal wall.

Follow with the **Back Muscles Stretch** (see figures 8.10 and 8.11). Again, take the time to feel the stretch deep along your spine.

UPPER BODY WORKOUT

The second phase of the intermediate exercise program focuses on working your neck and shoulder muscles with exercises from chapter 9. Start this phase by practicing the **Neck Flexion Exercise** (see figures 9.1 and 9.2) with 10 repetitions. Take your time during this exercise to feel the front of the neck muscles working.

Then move on and exercise the back of your neck with 10 repetitions of the **Neck Extension Exercise** (see figures 9.3 and 9.4) followed by 5 repetitions of the **Advanced Neck Extension Exercise** (see figures 9.5 and 9.6). Feel the exertions of the muscles at the back of your neck during this exercise.

Follow with the **Neck Half Rolls Exercise** (see figures 9.7 through 9.10) for 5 to 10 repetitions. Do not rush during this exercise. You want to feel your neck muscles contracting.

When done with the exercises, practice these neck stretches in the following order:

1. The **Back of the Neck Stretch** (see figures 9.22 and 9.23), gently and progressively stretching the back extensors, and the **Advanced Back of the Neck Stretch.**

2. The **Front of the Neck Stretch** (see figures 9.24 and 9.25), gently and progressively stretching the neck flexors, and the **Advanced Front of the Neck Stretch** (see figures 9.26 and 9.27).

3. The **Side of the Neck Stretch** (see figures 9.28 and 9.29), gently and progressively stretching the side neck muscles.

Now continue your exercise program by working your shoulders. Start with 5 repetitions of the **Shoulder Abduction Exercise** (see figures 9.16 and 9.17). Feel the rhomboid muscles working.

Next, work the **Shoulder Adduction Exercise** (see figures 9.18 and 9.19) with 5 repetitions. You can feel the pectoral muscles working.

Then proceed with 10 repetitions of the **Shoulder Circumduction (Circles) Exercise** (see figures 9.13 through 9.15). Move slowly because you want to feel every muscle that is worked as you perform this exercise.

Follow with the **Shoulder Shrug Exercise** (see figures 9.11 and 9.12). Start this exercise slowly to really feel the trapezius muscles working. Increase your rhythm as you proceed so that by the end of the twenty days you should be able to complete 20 repetitions.

Finally, work your trunk with 5 repetitions of the **Mid–Back Extension Exercise** (see figures 9.20 and 9.21). Do not rush through this exercise.

After finishing these exercises, follow with these shoulder stretches:

1. The **Back of the Shoulders Stretch** (see figures 9.30 and 9.31). Be gentle and do not jerk your arm. Strive to progressively develop the stretch.
2. The **Front of the Shoulders Stretch** (see figures 9.32 and 9.33), gently and progressively stretching your front shoulders.
3. The **Simultaneous Back of the Shoulders Stretch** (see figures 9.34 and 9.35), gently and progressively stretching the back of the shoulders.
4. The **Simultaneous Front of the Shoulders Stretch** (see figures 9.36 and 9.37), gently and progressively stretching the chest and arm muscles. Do not forget to end with the **Advanced Front of the Shoulders Stretch**.

LOWER BODY WORKOUT

Continue with the final phase of the intermediate program by working the exercises in chapter 10, which target your hips and legs. Start with the **Hip Flexion Exercise** (see figures 10.1 and 10.2) for 3 to 5 repetitions. Take your time during the early phases of this exercise so you can feel your hip flexor muscles working.

Follow with the **Hip Extension Exercise** (see figures 10.3 and 10.4) for 10 repetitions. Your hip extensor muscles are worked vigorously in this exercise. Make sure you reach the point where your knees lift off the floor.

Move on to the **Leg Squat Exercise** (see figures 10.5 and 10.6) with 10 repetitions. You should feel both your leg flexor and extensor muscles working when performing this exercise. Stay focused so that you squat all the way down, to where your buttocks touch your heels.

Next practice the **Leg Abduction Exercise** (see figures 10.11 and 10.12) with 10 repetitions followed by the **Leg Adduction Exercise** (see figures 10.13 and 10.14), also with 10 repetitions.

When done with these exercises, practice these hip stretches:

1. The **Back of the Hips Stretch** (see figures 10.15 and 10.16), gently and progressively stretching the back of the hips.
2. The **Front of the Hips Stretch** (see figures 10.17 and 10.18), gently and progressively stretching the front of the hips.

Finish the stretching phase of the intermediate program with these leg stretches:

1. The **Back of the Legs Stretch** (see figures 10.19 through 10.21), gently and progressively stretching the back of the legs.
2. The **Front of the Legs Stretch** (see figures 10.22 and 10.23), gently and progressively stretching the front of the legs.
3. The **Adductors of the Legs Stretch** (see figures 10.24 and 10.25), gently and progressively stretching the inner portion of the legs.
4. The **Abductors of the Legs Stretch** (see figures 10.26 and 10.27), gently and progressively stretching the outer portion of the legs.

Intermediate Exercise Program Chart

(20-minute Routine)

Order of Exercises	Exercise or Stretch	Repetitions	Time
1	Advanced Walking on the Spot Exercise	40–60	2 minutes
2	Scissor Feet Exercise	25	25 seconds
3	Abdominal Muscles Exercise	6	20 seconds
4	Advanced Abdominal Muscles Exercise	6	20 seconds
5	Back Muscles Exercise	10	50 seconds
6	Abdominal Muscles Stretch	1	15 seconds
7	Back Muscles Stretch	1	15 seconds
8	Neck Flexion Exercise	10	1 minute
9	Neck Extension Exercise	10	1 minute
10	Advanced Neck Extension Exercise	5	30 seconds
11	Neck Half Rolls Exercise	5–10	1 minute
12	Back of the Neck Stretch (and advanced version)	1	10 seconds
13	Front of the Neck Stretch (and advanced version)	1	10 seconds
14	Side of the Neck Stretch	1	20 seconds
15	Shoulder Abduction Exercise	5	1 minute
16	Shoulder Adduction Exercise	5	1 minute

(continued)

127

Intermediate Exercise Program Chart (continued)			
Order of Exercises	Exercise or Stretch	Repetitions	Time
17	Shoulder Circumduction (Circles) Exercise	10	15 seconds
18	Shoulder Shrug Exercise	20	15 seconds
19	Mid-Back Extension Exercise	5	20 seconds
20	Back of the Shoulders Stretch	1	20 seconds
21	Front of the Shoulders Stretch	1	20 seconds
22	Simultaneous Back of the Shoulders Stretch	1	10 seconds
23	Simultaneous Front of the Shoulders Stretch (and advanced version)	1	10 seconds
24	Hip Flexion Exercise	3–5	70 seconds
25	Hip Extension Exercise	10	70 seconds
26	Leg Squat Exercise	10	70 seconds
27	Leg Abduction Exercise	10	70 seconds
28	Leg Adduction Exercise	10	2½ minutes
29	Back of the Hips Stretch	1	15 seconds
30	Front of the Hips Stretch	1	15 seconds
31	Back of the Legs Stretch	1	25 seconds
32	Front of the Legs Stretch	1	25 seconds
33	Adductors of the Legs Stretch	1	25 seconds
34	Abductors of the Legs Stretch	1	25 seconds

14

The advanced exercise program is designed to maintain your body's musculature and flexibility. The level of fitness you have gained in the last month from practicing the beginning and intermediate programs has helped you to develop a strong seat and maintain flexibility when executing movement.

This advanced program starts with a warm-up, then moves on to exercises that will maintain strength in your back, front, torso, and leg muscles. As with the first two exercise routines, a chart covering all the exercises included in this advanced workout can be found at the end of this chapter. Use this chart along with the thumbnail figures shown on the tear sheets as a quick reference so you don't have to flip through the book while working out.

Finally, although this advanced program will help you maintain your fitness level, feel free to practice any of the other exercises presented in this book at any time in order to further develop your strength and flexibility.

WARM UP YOUR BODY

Start the advanced exercise program with some warm-up exercises from chapter 7. Begin with the **Advanced Walking on the Spot Exercise** (see figures 7.6 and 7.7) where you bring your knee up to the opposite side of your chest. Your pace should be to lift one knee every 2 seconds. Do 60 repetitions over the course of 1 minute.

Finish your warm-up with the **Scissor Feet Exercise** (see figures 7.8 through 7.10) doing 60 repetitions in 1 minute.

Maintenance of Your Back Core Muscles

The second phase of your advanced workout starts by working your back muscles. Practice the **General Extension Exercise** (see figures 11.1 and 11.2). Start gently and build up your endurance, holding the position for 20 seconds if you can. Repeat 5 times.

Follow with the **Back Muscles Stretch** (see figures 8.10 and 8.11) for 15 seconds.

Maintenance of Your Anterior Core Muscles

Next, you will work the core muscles on the front side of your body, which includes your neck, arms, abdomen, knees, hips, and legs. Begin with the **General Flexion Exercise** (see figures 11.3 and 11.4). Start gently and build up your endurance by holding the position for 30 seconds. Repeat 5 times.

Follow with the **Bridge Exercise** (see figures 11.10 through 11.12). Start gently and increase your endurance by holding this position for 8 seconds. Repeat 10 times.

Next move on to the **Knee Squeeze Exercise** (see figures 11.13 and 11.14). Repeat 10 times on each side, holding for 30 seconds each time.

Finally, stretch the core muscles you just worked with the **Abdominal Muscles Stretch** (see figures 8.8 and 8.9) for 15 seconds.

Maintenance of Your Torso Muscles

Move on to exercising your torso muscles with the **Twist Exercise** (see figures 11.5 through 11.7), building up to 30 repetitions. Follow with the **Advanced Twist Exercise** (see figures 11.8 and 11.9), where you lift your knees to the opposite side. Start gently and build up to 30 repetitions on each side.

Finish by stretching the torso muscles you just worked with the **Abdominal Muscles Stretch** (see figures 8.8 and 8.9) followed by the **Back Muscles Stretch** (see figures 8.10 and 8.11) for 15 seconds each.

MAINTENANCE OF YOUR
LEG MUSCLES

Finally, wrap up this exercise program with the **Advanced Leg Squat Exercise** (see figures 10.7 through 10.10). Start gently and build up to 25 repetitions in 2 minutes.

Finish with the **Back of the Legs Stretch** (see figures 10.19 through 10.21) and the **Front of the Legs Stretch** (see figures 10.22 and 10.23), holding each stretch for 15 seconds.

Advanced Exercise Program Chart
(15-Minute Routine)

Order of Exercises	Exercise or Stretch	Repetitions	Time
1	Advanced Walking on the Spot Exercise	60	1 minute
2	Scissor Feet Exercise	60	1 minute
3	General Extension Exercise	5	1 minute, 40 seconds
4	Back Muscles Stretch	1	15 seconds
5	General Flexion Exercise	5	2½ minutes
6	Bridge Exercise	10	1 minute, 20 seconds
7	Knee Squeeze Exercise	10 (per side)	5 minutes (per side)
8	Abdominal Muscles Stretch	1	15 seconds
9	Twist Exercise	30	1 minute
10	Advanced Twist Exercise	30	1 minute
11	Abdominal Muscles Stretch	1	15 seconds
12	Back Muscles Stretch	1	15 seconds
13	Advanced Leg Squat Exercise	25	2 minutes
14	Back of the Legs Stretch	1	15 seconds
15	Front of the Legs Stretch	1	15 seconds

15

People who have weak core muscles, imbalanced muscle tone, poor posture, and/or excessive weight might experience some back muscle soreness in the early aspects of their exercise routine. This is a natural response from the muscles to the new workload put on them. That is why I recommend you go easy in the early stages of your exercise program. Please focus on the quality of your movements rather than the quantity. As you develop your core muscles, you will be able to increase the amount of repetitions considerably by the second week, and by the end of the month you will be able to achieve the recommended number of repetitions.

However, when starting a new exercise regimen, and sometimes during the course of a program, your body might reveal one or more sore areas. This chapter addresses some of the most common issues you may face. But if you experience recurring problems, this material is not intended to replace the advice of a trained physician. When in doubt, please consult your doctor. When your doctor gives you the okay, you may resume practicing the exercises presented in this book.

SPINE AND LIMB SORENESS

When starting to exercise, stretching is the best way to test your body's capacity for handling stress on its muscles. If you're not sure about your ability to perform any particular exercise, first practice its corresponding stretch. If you feel soreness or pain during the stretch, then it's likely your skeleton is not properly aligned. As a matter of fact, if you experience spine or limb soreness during or after any of the exercises presented in this book, then you should consult your doctor, or even better, a chiropractor or osteopath.

Some examples of muscle stress include neck pinch, back and lower-back pinch, and sciatica. (*Sciatica* is a condition in which pain extends from your hip and down your leg; it is caused by a protruding vertebral disk that is pressing on the roots of the sciatic nerve.)

If any part of your spine (meaning your vertebrae) is not properly aligned, then this will cause the muscles, ligaments, and fascia layers in that area to tense up. This condition of misaligned vertebrae is referred to as a *vertebral subluxation*.

The muscles and fascia layers that attach to both sides of the actual subluxation will contract both as a compensatory and as a safety mechanism to prevent further damage to that area. If you feel any pain in your spine from these exercises, then get your spine checked by a trained professional in order to restore proper mobility and range of motion between each of your vertebra.

SHOULDER SORENESS

Sometimes a rider might feel soreness at the back of his shoulder(s). This discomfort is often related to the rotator cuff muscle group, which is made up of the supraspinatus, the infraspinatus, and the subscapularis muscles. The rotator cuff muscle group is responsible for securing the shoulder joint and for initiating the early movement of the arm's abduction. The deltoid muscle overlaps the shoulder joint and is responsible for most of the arm's abduction movement.

Sudden jolting to the arm can cause any of the muscles in the rotator cuff group to become strained and sore. Unfortunately, if pain within the rotator cuff muscle group continues or worsens, then it can lead to a more severe condition called *frozen shoulder*. This condition occurs when a muscle of the rotator cuff group *atrophies* (shrinks or weakens), causing severe restriction of movement and pain.

The best prevention against straining your rotator cuff muscles is to make sure they are in good shape. The Shoulder Circumduction (Circles) Exercise presented in chapter 9 is a good exercise for strengthening the rotator cuff muscle group. However, the Figure Eight Exercise (see page 135) is specifically designed to strengthen your rotator cuff muscle group, so if you begin to feel any soreness in your shoulders, then add this to your exercise program.

FIGURE EIGHT EXERCISE

The Figure Eight Exercise gets its name from the figure that your active hand makes during the exercise. By active, I mean the hand that is holding a small weight, such as a can of soda or peas, or a small dumbbell, if available. This particular figure eight movement allows you to exercise each of the three muscles involved in your rotator cuff muscle group. Regular practice of this exercise will keep this muscle group well toned and prevent the risk of injury.

Starting Position

You need to incorporate a chair or table to assist you with the Figure Eight Exercise. You also need a can of soda (a can of vegetables works, too). This exercise is done from a standing position, with your body leaning forward over a chair or table, as shown in figure 15.1.

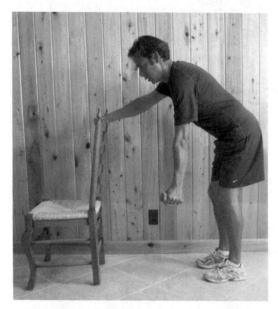

Figure 15.1 Figure Eight Exercise, starting position.

The Exercise

Start the exercise by taking a deep breath as you grab the soda can from the chair or table. Then, as you exhale, start moving your arm in a circle to the left, followed right away by another circle to the right, as if you were forming a figure eight in the air, as shown in figures 15.2 and 15.3.

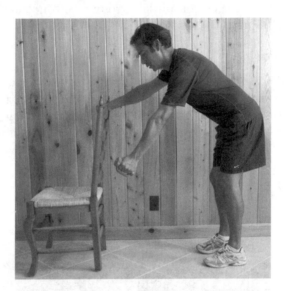

Figure 15.2 Figure Eight Exercise, circling to the left.

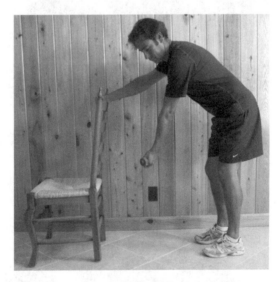

Figure 15.3 Figure Eight Exercise, circling to the right.

Repeat the figure eight movement 12 times with each arm. Do not rush. You should perform this exercise *slowly* in order to exercise all the rotator cuff muscles.

LEG CRAMPING

Many riders get calf or foot cramps during riding or shortly afterward. This is due to a lack of oxygen in the leg muscles. Performing the Leg Cramp Stretch immediately after cramping begins will help minimize the cramp's duration.

LEG CRAMP STRETCH

Starting Position

This stretch is best performed when sitting on your bed (or tack trunk if you're at the barn). Bring one leg up by bending your knee and resting your foot on the bed or tack trunk, as shown in figure 15.4.

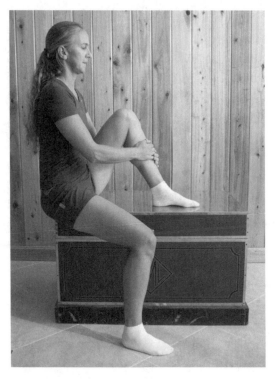

Figure 15.4 Leg Cramp Stretch,
starting position.

The Stretch

To begin the stretch, lock your fingers together around the ball of your foot and pull your foot up and toward your body until you reach an easy stretch, as shown in figure 15.5. For more efficiency, contract your shin muscles at the same time as you perform the stretch.

Hold the stretch 5 to 10 seconds or until the cramp disappears. Then consider pulling some more until you reach the deeper stretch. Feel your muscles relaxing. Then release the stretch to the starting position and repeat the exercise 2 to 3 times.

If you are subject to regular episodes of leg cramping, or other muscle cramping, please consult your doctor.

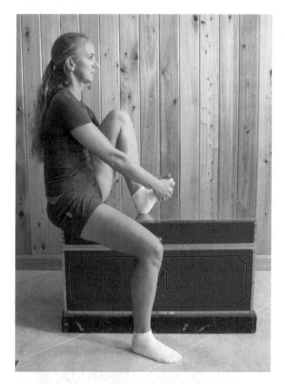

Figure 15.5 Leg Cramp Stretch,
ending position.

16

This book has given you a deeper understanding of the important role the core muscles play in postural awareness and healthy movement. The fitness of these particular muscles is vital to riders who want to achieve their best riding performance.

Written in a style that makes it easy to understand, this book has provided you with three unique and accessible programs of exercises and stretches designed to help you develop your core muscle for a better seat. No equipment is required, allowing you to practice any of these programs anywhere and at any time. Each program helps you progressively build your strength and enables you to reach your best riding fitness in a short period of time and to maintain this fitness level. I know this book will serve you well.

Enjoy your newfound awareness!

APPENDIX

SUGGESTED READINGS

The titles presented here are additional sources of information that will complement the material covered in this book. I encourage you to find time to read these important materials. Let them influence you as alternative approaches and methods to care for you and your animal in a gentle and loving way.

BOOKS

Anderson, Bob, *Stretching, 20th Anniversary Revised Edition*, Shelter Publications, 2000.

Budiansky, Stephen, *The Nature of Horses: Exploring Equine Evolution, Intelligence, and Behavior*, The Free Press, 1997.

Hourdebaigt, Jean-Pierre, LMT, *Equine Massage: A Practical Guide, Second Edition*, John Wiley & Sons, 2007.

Jacob, Stanley W., Clarice Ashworth Francone, and Walter J. Lossow, *Structure and Function in Man*, W B Saunders Company, 1982.

Myers, Thomas W., *Anatomy Trains: Myofascial Meridians for Manual and Movement Therapists*, Churchill Livingstone, 2001.

Southmayd, William, *Sport Health: The Complete Book of Athletic Injuries*, Quick Fox, 1981.

von Dietze, Susanne, *Balance in Movement: The Seat of the Rider*, Trafalgar Square Publishing, 1999.

INDEX

ABOUT THE AUTHOR

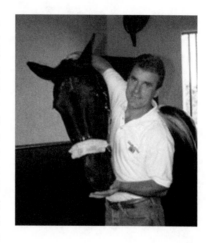

Born in the south of France, Jean-Pierre Hourdebaigt (pronounced Hoo-da-bay) moved to Canada in 1981 where he continued a generations-old family practice of natural healing. In 1983, after graduating at the top of his class from the Canadian College of Massage and Hydrotherapy, he began a successful career as a Registered Massage Therapist treating athletes and dignitaries from around the world. Jean-Pierre's talented, skilled hands have greatly improved the lives of people who sustained injuries from motor vehicle and sports-related accidents. His experience in working with top Canadian athletes, sports medicine doctors, and physical therapists enhanced his knowledge of physical fitness, especially regarding how to develop and maintain peak fitness.

For years, Jean-Pierre has applied his knowledge of massage therapy to horses, dogs, and cats, managing hundreds of animals. It was his empathy and passion for animals that led him to research and develop material related to the massage of animals.

In 2001, Jean-Pierre moved to Wellington, Florida, to expand his equine and canine practice and to continue his research on new massage techniques for conditions such as Equine Temporomandibular Dysfunction Syndrome (ETDS) and for the study of equine muscular compensation. He continues to treat human athletes, too. While assisting riders of all levels and disciplines, he became aware of the common problems inherent in the sport of riding. Feedback from many clients helped him better understand the nature of the musculoskeletal injuries seen in the sport. As a result, Jean-Pierre developed a training program to assist riders in improving their core fitness in order to avoid most riding-related injuries.

For questions or commentary, Jean-Pierre Hourdebaigt can be reached through his web site, www.massageawareness.com.

ABOUT MASSAGE AWARENESS

Jean-Pierre Hourdebaigt created his company, Massage Awareness Incorporated (MAInc.), in order to pass on his massage expertise and thereby reach more people. His company's mission statement follows: Massage Awareness, Inc. is devoted to the education of people in the art and application of massage using the **Massage Awareness Method**, so they can actively participate in a natural way in the fitness and well-being of their animal companion.

Jean-Pierre has applied European techniques and his knowledge of massage therapy to horses, dogs, and cats, managing thousands of animals over the years. His empathy and compassion for animals allows him to communicate with them on a special level. This passion led him to develop the Massage Awareness Method, which uses massage techniques to enhance the performance and quality of life of animals by increasing flexibility, reducing stiffness, improving attitude, and shortening recovery time from injury. A side benefit is that it makes people feel really good about the care they are providing for their animals. Jean-Pierre has found that *"the action of giving a massage provides positive feedback for the person on the musculoskeletal fitness of their animal and enhances a closer relationship between pet and owner."*

Jean-Pierre's caring and holistic approach, massage therapy expertise, and teaching experience have enabled animal lovers to develop and enjoy healthier, happier, more productive relationships with their equine and canine friends. He has taught animal lovers with a variety of backgrounds worldwide, including: veterinarians and veterinary technicians; physiotherapists; massage therapists; farriers; breeders; trainers; competitive and recreational horseback riders; and dog owners, groomers, handlers, obedience and agility competitors; and owners and trainers of seeing-eye dogs. Attendees have come away from his seminars feeling comfortable and confident in applying the Massage Awareness Method to help their animals.

Today, Jean-Pierre resides in Florida where he is continuing his work in human and animal massage therapy. He offers educational seminars, practical training sessions, and private tutoring to those who want to learn animal massage. He travels around the world to share his immense knowledge and love of animals.

Books

Because of his unique talents and efforts in helping animals with massage, Jean-Pierre has been interviewed by a number of TV and radio shows, and written about in newspapers and magazines throughout Canada and the United States. In January 1997, he wrote his first book, *Equine Massage: A Practical Guide* (Howell Book House, New York), for horse enthusiasts around the world. Jean-Pierre fully revised and updated the second edition of this book in 2007.

His second book, *Canine Massage: A Practical Guide* (Howell Book House, New York), was nominated for an award at the 1999 Writing Competition of the Dog Writer's Association of America (DWAA) in the Care and Health Book Division.

Self-Published Books

Jean-Pierre has also self-published several interesting books, which are available for purchase from www.massageawareness.com, including:

1. *Equine Muscular Anatomy and Kinesiology*
   This book provides an extensive overview of more than 115 important muscles and corresponding fasciae in the equine muscular system. For each muscle, you are given the following information: location, origin tendon, point insertion, tendon blood supply (veins and arteries), nerve supply, and action. A section on equine kinesiology is also offered. This knowledge of the equine musculature coupled with your massage skills will directly affect the quality of your performance, which benefits your horse.

2. *ETDS: Equine Temporomandibular Dysfunction Syndrome*
   Poor performance of the temporomandibular joint will result in poor *mastication* (chewing) and possible digestive complications. A healthy temporomandibular joint is necessary for good contact at the bit, enabling proper performance of the equine athlete and helping the rider to delicately direct the horse. Massage treatment for Equine Temporomandibular Dysfunction Syndrome (ETDS) is a noninvasive approach that works in harmony with the horse. It allows you to assess muscle tone and stiffness, find imbalances, and help correct these imbalances. This book provides all the information you need to know on the topic. Early detection of this condition helps you maximize your animal's well being and save on recovery time, as well as save money that you would have spent on treatment for your horse.

3. *Equine Muscular Compensation, a Study*

The popularity of equestrian sports has triggered a renewed interest in the study of equine locomotion and training techniques. This book gives you a clear picture of the equine muscular compensation phenomenon, including how it occurs, the structures involved, and how to recognize its symptoms. This knowledge will help you better understand how your horse moves and will help you make the right decisions to improve the wellness and fitness of your equine friend.

4. *Equine Myofascial Massage, Foundation Course*

Myofascial therapy is one of the most important evolutions in alternative medicine. Equine myofascial massage specializes in the myofascial system of the body, which includes fascial layers, fascial bands, retinaculum, ligaments, and tendons. This massage therapy relieves any alterations sustained during injury and helps to maintain optimal flexibility of the fascia system. It also enhances the performance, flexibility, rehabilitation, and wellness of the equine athlete. This book teaches you everything you need and want to know about equine myofascial massage.

CANINE-RELATED BOOKS

Jean-Pierre's passion for dogs has led him to publish canine massage books as well, including:

1. *Canine Muscular Anatomy and Kinesiology*
2. *Canine Muscular Compensation, a Study*
3. *Canine Myofascial Massage, Foundation Course*

You will also find DVDs, laminated muscle charts, stress point location posters, and more on the Massage Awareness Web site.

CONTACT INFORMATION

If you wish to meet Jean-Pierre at his company's location or if you wish to have him come to yours, you can contact him directly through his Web site, www.massageawareness.com, for more details.

Jean-Pierre is constantly researching and writing on new, important topics related to the health and benefit of animals.

TAKE-ALONG EXERCISE GUIDES

Now you can do your exercises anywhere! This fold-out insert details both the Intermediate Exercise Program and the Advanced Exercise Program from chapters 13 and 14. Tear out the routine you need and take it with you as a quick reference when you're away from home.

The exercises are presented in the same order as they are in the chapters. To guide you through each routine, you'll find photos that walk you through each exercise step, along with the number of repetitions you should do and approximately how long each exercise will take.

19. Shoulder Shrug Exercise—20 repetitions (15 seconds)

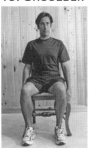 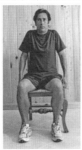

20. Mid-Back Extension Exercise—5 repetitions (20 seconds)

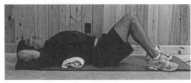 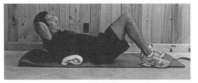

21. Back of the Shoulders Stretch—20 seconds

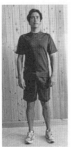 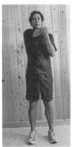

22. Front of the Shoulders Stretch—20 seconds

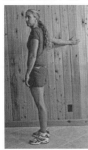 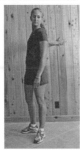

23. SIMULTANEOUS BACK OF THE SHOULDERS STRETCH—10 SECONDS

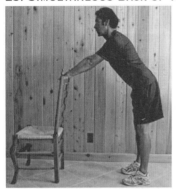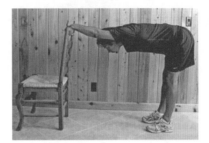

24. SIMULTANEOUS FRONT OF THE SHOULDERS STRETCH—10 SECONDS

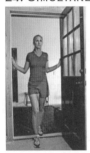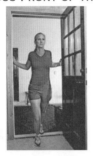

25. HIP FLEXION EXERCISE—3 TO 5 REPETITIONS (1 MINUTE, 10 SECONDS)

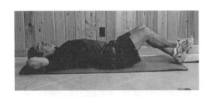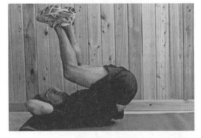

26. HIP EXTENSION EXERCISE—10 REPETITIONS (1 MINUTE, 10 SECONDS)

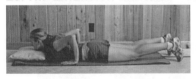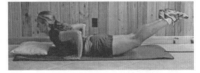

ADVANCED EXERCISE PROGRAM

1. ADVANCED WALKING ON THE SPOT EXERCISE—60 REPETITIONS (1 MINUTE)

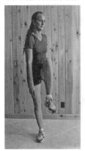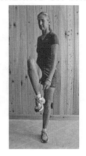

2. SCISSOR FEET EXERCISE—60 REPETITIONS (1 MINUTE)

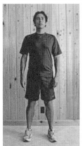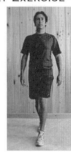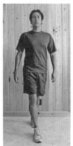

3. GENERAL EXTENSION EXERCISE—5 REPETITIONS (1 MINUTE, 40 SECONDS)

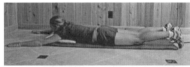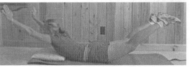

4. BACK MUSCLES STRETCH—15 SECONDS

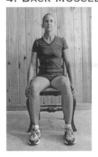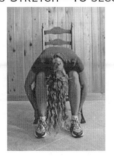

5. General Flexion Exercise—5 repetitions (2 minutes, 30 seconds)

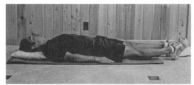 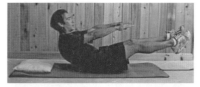

6. Bridge Exercise—10 repetitions (1 minute, 20 seconds)

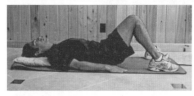 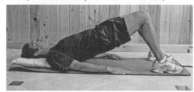

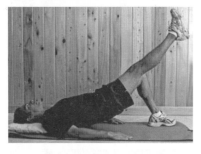

7. Knee Squeeze Exercise—10 repetitions per side (3 to 5 minutes per side)

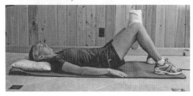 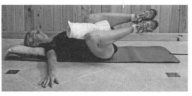

8. Abdominal Muscles Stretch—15 seconds

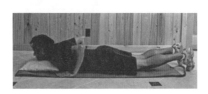 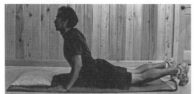